ELECTRO
ACUPUNCTURE
HANDBOOK

ELECTRO
ACUPUNCTURE
HANDBOOK
for musculoskeletal problems

Stephen Lee BA MBAcC MRCHM

Practising acupuncturist and herbalist

Foreword by

David Mayor MA BAc MBAcC

Honorary member AACP, Acupuncture practitioner and
Visiting Fellow (Physiotherapy), University of Hertfordshire, UK

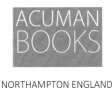

NORTHAMPTON ENGLAND

First published in 2018
by Acuman Books
136 Birchfield Road
Northampton NN1 4RH, UK

First published 2017
    Reprinted 2020, 2021, 2024

ISBN 978-1-9996152-0-8

The contents and techniques outlined in this book are intended as a resource and guide for trained practitioners of acupuncture. It is not intended as a substitute for such training. While every effort has been made to include cautions with regard to electro-acupuncture treatment, the author cannot accept responsibility for any treatment advice or information offered.

Design, layout and illustration - Dragonwerk Graphics
Printed by Mixam

Contents

Foreword

I have known Stephen Lee since we were both students at JR Worsley's College of Traditional Acupuncture in Leamington Spa in the early 1980s. We would meet quite regularly in London for the point location training sessions held at the Ladbroke Grove home of the late and wonderful Madeleine Molder, but then our paths diverged, and at that stage I don't think either of us imagined that they would come together again in the future.

My own interest in electroacupuncture (EA) dates back to before the time we trained, and I began to teach, very tentatively, in 1996, the same year that I started work on my own textbook on EA, work that took me 11 painstaking years to complete. It took a little longer before Stephen began to teach, and a further 10 years before he felt ready to produce this, his first acupuncture textbook.

It is now over a decade since my own book was published, and it is quite out of date – for instance the number of studies on 'electroacupuncture' listed in PubMed as published in the 50 years up to the end of 2007 was less than 2000; since then, numbers have increased dramatically, with coming up to 3000 appearing in the last decade alone. It is thus almost impossible for anyone to do today what I attempted and explore all the information that is out there on EA. Although I believe my own book is still a useful place to start, there is a real need for more focused and practical books such as Stephen's.

While writing this foreword, I was surprised to find there are a few recent EA books listed on Amazon, including one from Korea and another from Brazil on microcurrent EA. But Stephen's is the most appropriate for anyone wanting to learn more about how to actually use EA for musculoskeletal conditions – the field in which it is most frequently applied.

The book is eminently readable, not least because of the clarity of Stephen's own illustrations. He does not pontificate or throw 'scientific' or 'traditional' theories about unnecessarily, is humble about what he doesn't know and when EA cannot help, and not wedded to rigid ideas about how treatment should be applied. Nonetheless, he gives clear and careful guidelines on the usual sorts of conditions acupuncturists are likely to meet in their practice, including some quite difficult ones. The cases he presents are both informative and inspirational.

I can certainly say I have learned a lot from reading his book, as I did from sitting in the back row at one of his courses. His extensive experience in treating elderly patients has also confirmed my own observations – that the notion that strong EA may be 'draining' for deficient patients is really a 'self-perpetuating myth' (p 19).

In particular, I like the way Stephen explains how EA works for musculoskeletal problems in terms of the movements of *qi* and blood and tissue healing, and his resultant emphasis on muscle palpation (rather than laboriously naming muscles). Although he pays passing homage to the mammoth body of Chinese research on the neurophysiology of EA for pain, spearheaded by Han Jisheng's group in Beijing since the 1970s, he is wise enough to question whether this should always determine the stimulation frequencies we should use in practice. As a result, over the years his approach in this regard has evolved, as has my own. We may not always agree (as in where clips should be attached to the needles, for example), but such differences can lead to friendly debate rather than bristly stand-offs, and we are both willing to learn from each other.

All in all, this is a book I can heartily recommend, both as a complement to my own somewhat magisterial tome and as a good and useful stand-alone introduction to the use of EA for musculo-skeletal problems.

2018

David Mayor MA BAc MBAcC
Acupuncture practitioner
Honorary member AACP
Visiting Fellow (Physiotherapy)
University of Hertfordshire, UK

Preface

I have to confess that I tend to err on the anti-technological end of the spectrum so it is somewhat ironic that I am sitting here on my computer writing a book about electroacupuncture (EA). My interest in EA is simply the result of a real desire to treat patients successfully. What I've discovered over the last 30 years is that EA is much more effective for musculoskeletal problems, generally speaking, than manual acupuncture (MA). I know this because patients have told me.

When I purchased my first EA machine in the early 1980s there was very little information available on how to use it. I therefore set about developing my own methods and understanding. In the beginning I saw things very much from a TCM perspective in terms of the meridians, zang fu, pathogenic factors etc. As I became more familiar with musculoskeletal acupuncture and its success in treating muscles and joints, I began to combine EA with these treatments which made them even more effective. Developing these techniques has been a long process but I now feel I have something worth sharing with the acupuncture community at large.

I first wrote an article on EA in 2008 which was published in the *European Journal of Oriental Medicine* (Lee 2008) and then the revised version appeared in *The Journal of Chinese Medicine* (Lee 2010). Since then I have presented this material at a number of workshops, and met several practitioners, some working in NHS pain clinics, who have found the techniques to be very effective. The material from these articles and workshops has culminated in the book you are now holding. I hope you find it a useful guide to this intriguing subject.

2018   Stephen Lee

Acknowledgements

First I would like to thank my teachers at the College of Traditional Acupuncture at Leamington Spa who introduced me to the world of acupuncture and gave me the confidence to practise. I am also grateful to the gang of four - Vivienne Brown, Peter Deadman, Giovanni Maciocia and Julian Scott - who came back from China in the early 80s and introduced us all to the treasure house of TCM which grounded my practice. I appreciated the time I spent with Dr Gu, Dr Wu and Dr Shen in Nanjing in 1987; they showed me how TCM was applied in a hospital setting with humour and compassion.

It was David Legge who prompted my interest in the musculoskeletal aspects of the body; and Kevin Young and Tony Brewer who taught me how to use acupuncture to treat musculoskeletal problems.

David Mayor's support has been invaluable, in particular through his seminars and the advice he has given me regarding my teaching and writing about EA. And I will always be grateful to Angela Hicks for encouraging me to continue with my teaching when my confidence wavered. Dominic Rushmore, my fellow acupuncturist and friend, has patiently schooled me in the basics of electrical theory on our many morning walks round the local park.

I would like to thank Sandie George and my daughter Catherine Lee for their advice on scientific matters and all my diligent proofreaders, Eva Barton, Kathy Barton, Maria Lee and Tim Stillwell, for their helpful input.

Key

ashi   is the Chinese word to denote a point of tenderness felt by a patient on palpation. The words tenderness, soreness and ashi have been used interchangeably through-out the book to refer to these points.

capitals When capitals are used for organ names or body fluids (e.g. Liver, Blood) the terms refer to TCM concepts.

cun   traditional measurement in Chinese medicine equivalent to the width of the patient's thumb joint

EA   electroacupuncture

ES   electrical stimulation

EF   electric field

DD   dense/disperse

HF   high frequency

LF   low frequency

L3(R)   3rd lumbar vertebra on the right hand side

MA   manual acupuncture

T8(L)   thoracic vertebra on the left hand side

TCM   traditional Chinese medicine

QL   quadratus lumborum

●   When a black dot appears on its own in an illustration it signifies an ashi point and/or possible treatment point.

✕   location of MA needle

When dots and lines are combined, the dots represent the insertion points of the needles in the body, the thin lines represent the wires.

When thick and thin lines are combined, the medium lines are the needle shafts, the thick lines are the needle handles, the thin lines represent the wires.

Introduction

I suspect that EA is not widely used in our profession simply because, being a relatively new addition to Chinese medicine, our knowledge of it is limited. Consequently it is not taught in any significant depth and practitioners do not all have the confidence to apply EA successfully. I meet many people who have bought EA machines but don't know how to use them. This book is a response to this situation and written in the hope that this valuable tool will be used more widely in future. It may also initiate a dialogue with practitioners of other disciplines who use EA so that we can gather a broader body of knowledge on the subject. It should be noted that none of the information presented here is set in stone and should be seen as work in progress.

From a traditional Chinese medical perspective my understanding is that EA moves stagnation of qi and Blood and thus normalises the functioning of dysfunctional muscles and joints thereby relieving pain. I find EA is particularly useful for treating chronic musculoskeletal problems such as osteoarthritis of the hip or frozen shoulder, where manual acupuncture and other physical therapies have been ineffective. EA is also very effective at healing scar tissue.

For many traditionalists in the acupuncture profession, EA is considered superfluous to an already complete art - a gross technological intrusion into the subtle energies of the body. But so, of course, is a hip replacement, which I imagine nobody would refuse if faced with the prospect of long term chronic pain. This view ignores the rich and fascinating connections and articulations of the muscles, tendons, ligaments and fascia. This book is therefore primarily presented from a musculoskeletal point of view rather than a TCM perspective. At the same time I would insist that EA treatment is most effective when the underlying constitutional disharmonies of a person are addressed.

I think that sometimes the practice of Chinese medicine in the west has become too holistic, the belief being that if we can address a person's overall disharmony we can affect any musculoskeletal problems successfully. It is easy to think that a particular organ or meridian is the primary culprit in any problem but it may be that a particular muscle group is the real cause of the problem. We know from western psychological ideas that deep unresolved emotions, stress and trauma can be held in the muscles of the body in the same way that Chinese medicine recognises that psychological problems can affect the organ systems. It is not unreasonable to think that the stagnation of Blood caused by chronic tightness in large muscle groups could impede the overall circulation of blood as much as Liver stasis. So it might follow that by addressing a particular muscle group we can bring the whole system back into harmony both on a physical and psychological level.

Chronic musculoskeletal problems can be very distressing and ultimately debilitating, so it would be counterproductive not to give them the same degree of significance as internal problems. It is also worth noting that it is primarily for musculoskeletal problems that people seek acupuncture.

I think there is a tendency for traditional acupuncturists to believe that using electricity is unnatural or possibly cheating, like Vermeer using lenses and mirrors to paint his masterpieces (which he probably did). I however would like to challenge this notion and argue that electricity is an entirely natural healing modality that is very effective where manual acupuncture fails. It is very easy to be misled into thinking that the body is a biological system built on bones articulated by muscles and ligaments, and containing organs that perform a plethora of functions, such as producing blood or circulating body fluids. The truth is that we are as electrical as we are biochemical: not a thought, movement, heartbeat, visual or auditory perception can occur without electricity. We are beings animated by electricity. Western medicine has utilised electricity to keep hearts beating with pacemakers; to help people hear with cochlear implants, and to control Parkinson's tremors with deep brain electrical stimulation. It is perfectly reasonable for us to utilise electricity to enhance our acupuncture treatments.

The conditions covered in this book are some of the most common problems that I see in my clinic and by no means the only conditions that can be treated with EA. Once the general principles of EA are grasped then of course they can be applied to many other musculoskeletal problems.

Electricity

It's hard to imagine how exciting it must have been to discover not only how to generate electricity but also the effects of electricity on living organisms. In 1781 Luigi Galvani, an Italian physician, physicist, biologist and philosopher, discovered he could make the muscles of a dead frog twitch by applying electricity. He must have believed that he had discovered the very force that animates life itself. In 1759, John Wesley, the founder of the Methodist church, claimed that electricity 'was the spirit of God manifest'. He went on to use electrical therapy in the free clinics he established to treat the poor. He also wrote a book with the charming and intriguing title, 'The Desideratum: or, electricity made plain and useful by a lover of mankind and common sense'. Wesley used electricity to treat sciatica, headaches, gout and kidney stones.

This was not the first time that electricity had been used to treat health problems; there is evidence that the Egyptians used electric fish, particularly the Nile catfish (malapterurus electricus) to treat various conditions in 2500BC. Hippocrates, too, is said to have used electric fish as a therapy. One imagines that electric fish therapy was very impractical to administer and possibly unpleasant to receive which is probably why it never caught on. It was not until the 18th century and the discovery of how to generate and store electricity in a controlled manner that electrotherapy really took off.

The use of electricity for medical purposes was facilitated by the invention of the Leyden jar in 1745 by Ewald G. von Kleist and Pieter van Musschenbroek as it enabled static electricity to be stored and discharged as needed. The development of batteries coupled with experimental procedures on humans and animals by electrotherapy pioneers such as Giovanni Aldini, Alexandro Volta, Johann Krüger and Christian Kratzenstein meant that electrical therapy became more popular.

In 1752 Benjamin Franklin used electricity to treat a neighbour's frozen shoulder and a number of women for convulsions. In Japan in 1764 Gennai Hiraga was using electricity to stimulate acupuncture needles to treat muscle spasm and paralysis. In 1768 we see the first electrical therapy apparatus installed in a

London hospital. In 1812 John Birch was using electricity to treat non-union tibial fractures at St Thomas's Hospital. It was not until 1823 that the word 'electropuncture' was coined by Jean-Baptiste Sarlandière, a French anatomist and physiologist, who used EA to treat asthma, colic, gout, migraines, 'nervous affliction', paralysis and rheumatism. His patients apparently found the experience so 'delicious' that 'they begged (him) to continue forever'! (cited in Mayor 2007). The Victorians embraced electrotherapy with all sorts of electrical devices to treat a variety of ailments.

In view of electrotherapy's long history there is no reason not to utilise it in order to help our patients. We should adopt the pragmatism of the Chinese and use what works rather than limiting ourselves to a particular ideological or theoretical model.

Keown postulated in *The Spark in the Machine* (2014) that acupuncture is a process of generating micro-electric currents through the highly conductive fascia of the body. Enhancing this process using EA makes logical sense.

As traditional acupuncturists, we are very familiar with the concept of qi as an invisible and elusive substance. Electricity is in many ways very similar to the concept of qi, in that it is an invisible substance that circulates throughout the body, initiating and influencing its many functions. If everything in the universe is a manifestation of qi, then electricity can be viewed as another such manifestation.

ELECTRICAL PRINCIPLES

In order to use EA confidently it is helpful to have an understanding of electricity. The term electricity covers a number of phenomena that are the result of the flow of electric charge including lightning, static electricity and the flow of electric current down a wire. Electric current results from the effect of electrical potential on charged particles (electrons).

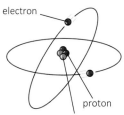

Fig. 1. 1

Electrons are wave-particles that orbit the nucleus of an atom. The nucleus consists of protons and neutrons (Fig. 1. 1). Current is the movement of charge and is measured in amperes (amps).

If the negative pole of a battery is connected to the positive pole with a wire, electrons start to flow along the wire from the negative pole to the positive (Fig. 1. 2). This happens because there is a potential difference in energy between the positive and negative poles of the battery, which is measured in volts (V). One of the properties of metals is that some of the electrons have a weaker bond to the nucleus than others allowing them to move from one atom to

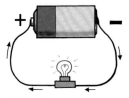

Fig. 1. 2

the next; it is this property that allows the electrical charge to move along the wire. This movement of charge in one direction is called direct current (DC). DC is also called monophasic current. If DC current were used for EA it could cause electrolysis (and even corrosion) of the needles at the point of insertion. Electrolysis is the chemical process caused by the flow of electrical current through conductive fluids.

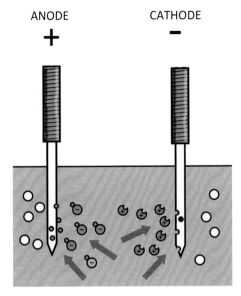

ANODE   CATHODE

+   −

Fig. 1. 3

ALTERNATING CURRENT

To avoid the problem of electrolysis, EA machines are designed to deliver alternating current (AC), also known as biphasic current, as the flow of electrical charge continuously alternates, moving first in one direction and then the other. The same type of current is used in our domestic electricity supply. The number of times that the current alternates per second is called frequency and is measured in hertz (Hz). So 20 hertz indicates that the electricity changes direction 20 times per second. A complete movement of current in one direction and then the other is referred to as a cycle. With high frequencies the electrons may only move a short distance before changing direction.

DURING TREATMENT

Let's look at what occurs to the movement of electrical current during an EA treatment. Electricity, carried by the electrons, first moves down the wire from the machine to a needle. From here, the flow of electricity continues by different means. Because the human body is not made of metal, electrons are not

- **Volts (V)** measure the **potential energy** e.g. the energy in a battery

- **Amperes (amps)** measure the **current**, the strength of delivery of the electricity

- **Hertz (Hz)** measure the **frequency** which is the number of times that the electricity with **alternating current** changes direction per second. One backwards and one forwards movement is called a **cycle**

free to flow from atom to atom, but instead the current utilises ions (ie positively and negatively charged atoms or molecules) suspended in body fluids. Fluids containing ions are called electrolytes.

A positively charged ion (cation) has one or more electrons missing and a negatively charged ion (anion) has one or more extra electrons. Because opposite charges attract, the cations move towards the cathode and the anions move towards the anode (Fig. 1. 3). Due to the alternating nature of AC, at any given moment during EA treatment, one of each pair of needles will be positively charged and the other negatively charged causing the electricity to move backwards and forwards through the electrolyte.

Because with AC the current can rapidly change direction (determined by the frequency setting on the EA machine), the migration of ions to the positively or negatively charged needle can be short-lived meaning that the exchange of electrons at the needles is minimal.

At high frequencies it may be that the ions are oscillating on the spot giving the surrounding tissues a vigorous massage at an atomic and molecular level.

WAVES

If electricity is passed through an oscilloscope, a visual representation of the electric current is produced in the form of waves. Figure 1. 4 shows an AC wave generated by an oscilloscope. The wave

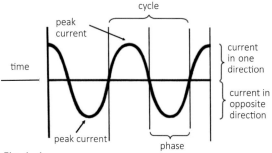

Fig. 1. 4

above the baseline represents the strength of the current as it moves in one direction at any given moment, and the wave below the line represents the strength of the current as it moves in the opposite direction. This vertical axis represents the amplitude i.e. the strength of the current which is adjusted using the intensity control on the EA machine. The wave above the line combined with the wave below the line is one cycle and is measured as 1Hz. The horizontal axis represents time.

The phase duration is the width of one wave and is measured in microseconds (μs). The shape of the wave represents how quickly or slowly the amplitude increases or decreases. If there is a sudden increase in the amplitude then the wave appears as a 'step' upwards or downwards from the baseline. If the increase and decrease is gradual it appears as a gradually inclining and declining line. If there is a pause between cycles this is called an interpulse (Fig. 1. 5).

Fig. 1. 6 shows a continuous square wave, an intermittent square wave and a dense-disperse (DD) wave.

HABITUATION

If the body is stimulated with one continuous frequency it tends to become used to it and stops responding; this is known as habituation. In order to avoid this, the electrical signal can be adjusted to produce patterns of varying frequency, which is

referred to as dense-disperse stimulation. EA machines can be set so that they deliver two frequencies one followed by the other (see last image in Fig. 1 .6). Examples of this would be settings of 150Hz and 50 Hz, or 90Hz and 30Hz. This means that the machine might deliver 90Hz for a couple of seconds followed by 30Hz for another couple of seconds. If DD is selected on my machine the second frequency is automatically set to a third of the first frequency selected e.g. if it is set on DD at 100Hz the other frequency will be 33Hz.

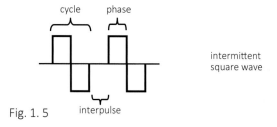

Fig. 1. 5

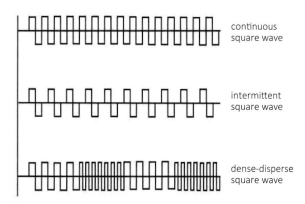

Fig. 1. 6

Electrical effects on the body

2

E A involves electrophysical, electrochemical and electrothermal phenomena (Cameron 2012). The body is a complex multifaceted system in which processes occur; on an electrical, chemical, cellular, organ, neural and musculoskeletal level. From electrical impulses relaying sensory information or initiating muscular contractions to neurons triggering a cascade of hormonal activity, electricity is fundamental to the body's many processes.

Ever since President Richard Nixon went to China in 1972 and witnessed an operation being performed using acupuncture anaesthesia, research has focused predominantly on how acupuncture, EA and electrotherapy controls pain by stimulating the body's own natural chemical painkillers. As a result of this, relatively little research has concentrated on the healing effects of electricity e.g. the restoration of normal muscle function or the healing of tissue.

A brief trawl of the literature will reveal a vast amount of research looking at the effects of electricity on the body; its breadth and depth are truly impressive. A full and detailed review is beyond the scope of this book, which is essentially a 'how to do it' book as opposed to a 'how does it work' book. However, I provide below a summary of the main areas of research to give the reader a flavour. This is by no means a complete or up to date review.

Much of today's practice of EA is the result of experimentation conducted in China post 1950 (Dharmananda 2002). Experiments conducted by Professor Ji-Sheng Han at the Beijing Medical University led to EA devices being used to provide pain relief for patients undergoing surgery. Professor Ji-Sheng Han found that for 11% of patients, EA alone was sufficient to provide adequate pain relief. It was misreported in the West that patients were routinely undergoing surgery in China with EA as the only form of pain relief. In reality it was frequently being used as an adjunct to other analgesics such as local anaesthesia and opiates. It was partly these misleading reports that caused a renewed interest in acupuncture and EA in the West. In China today EA is not used as a substitute for analgesia but rather a pre and post-operative treatment (Gyer, Michael and Tolson 2016).

Much of the research is focused on EA's ability to induce an analgesic effect both on the central (CNS) and peripheral nervous system (PNS) through influencing neurotransmitters and modulators (Hsieh *et al.* 2000; He 1987; Pomeranz, Cheng and Law 1977). Studies hypothesise that a number of signalling molecules are involved, such as endogenous opioid peptides, cholecystokinin octapeptides, noradrenaline, serotonin, dopamine, glutamate, γ-aminobutyric acid as well as other bioactive substances which may affect the CNS and PNS directly (Leung 2012; Yoo *et al.* 2011; Zhao 2008). Studies by Lin and Chen (2008) indicate that other systems are also involved in EA pain modulation including the hypothalamus-pituitary-adrenal axis, a division of the PNS called the autonomic nervous system and the descending inhibitory pathways (hypothalamus-periaqueductal grey area-raphe nucleus-spinal cord).

GATE CONTROL THEORY

The gate control theory, outlined by Melzack and Wall (1965), proposes that the transmission of pain is modulated at the level of the spinal cord.

This theory asserts that transmission of sensory information from a site of injury is carried along two types of nerve fibre: thin diameter nerve fibres which carry pain signals; and large diameter nerve fibres which carry non-nociceptive sensory information such as touch, pressure and vibration. These nerve fibres converge at a transmission cell and have a differential effect on the transmission cell's likelihood of firing and thus the likelihood of the signal reaching the brain. The thin nerve fibres increase the likelihood of the transmission cell firing whilst the thick nerve fibres decrease this likelihood. This is used to explain why rubbing an area after it has been hit tends to reduce pain sensation: with a higher proportion of large nerve fibres being stimulated, the number of pain signals transmitted by transmission cells is reduced.

The mechanism of action of transcutaneous electrical nerve stimulation (TENS) for chronic pain can also be explained using this theory; by stimulating more large diameter nerve fibres, pain transmission is reduced. TENS is a method of pain relief which uses conductive pads to transmit electrical impulses to the skin of the painful area; it has been recommended by physiotherapists for many years within both the NHS and private health services.

In 1967, Wall and Sweet found that 50% of their sample of patients experienced relief from chronic neurological pain when needles were used to deliver a relatively high frequency current (50-100Hz). The gate control theory suggests that this frequency stimulated the large diameter nerve fibres more than the thin ones thus "closing the gate" to pain transmission which, at the level of the spinal cord, involves endorphins, as well as non-opioid neurotransmitters such as gamma-aminobutyric acid (Bowsher 1998).

In 1967, Shealy and colleagues implanted electrodes into the spinal cord to relieve chronic pain; this procedure was the forerunner of modern day spinal (dorsal) stimulation therapy (Shealy *et al.* 1967).

In the early 1970s TENS was being use to predict whether individuals would be suitable for dorsal column stimulation therapy. This is a technique used in the management of certain chronic pain syndromes such as failed back surgery syndrome and complex regional pain syndrome: electrodes are surgically implanted in the posterior aspect of the spinal cord through which electricity is delivered to relieve the pain. When using TENS they realised that it could be used in its own right for other types of pain (Long 1974).

Psychological distraction or motivational techniques can also "close the gates" in the spinal cord thus reducing pain transmission.

ENDORPHIN THEORY

Endogenous opioids (beta-endorphins, enkephalins, endomorphins and dynorphins) occur naturally in the body and can both reduce pain sensations and produce feelings of euphoria. According to the endorphin theory, acupuncture reduces pain through the release of these chemicals. This hypothesis is supported by the findings of research carried out by Pomeranz and Chiu (1976). Rats were injected with naloxone, an opioid antagonist, which resulted in the analgesic effects of EA being blocked. Research using naloxone to investigate the role of endorphins in acupuncture analgesia has also been carried out in humans with similar effects (Mayer, Price and Rafii 1977).

Mayor (2007) asserted the current consensus to be as follows: low frequency (LF) EA stimulates the release of beta-endorphins, enkephalins and endomorphins (which act on mu- and delta-opioid receptors) whilst high frequency (HF) EA stimulates the release of dynorphins (which act on kappa-opioid receptors) and possibly triggers other non-opioid mechanisms as well.

Fei, Sun and Han (1988) studied the impact of EA on endogenous opioids and found different frequencies led to the release of different opioids. More specifically Guo *et al.* (1996) observed that low frequency EA (2Hz) increased the expression of enkephalin precursor proteins and high frequency (100Hz) led to the production of dynorphin precursors. Further, Chen & Han (1992) found that EA analgesia is mediated by different opioid receptors depending on EA frequency. Han *et al.* (1999) later found that low (2Hz) but not high frequency (100Hz) EA analgesia was mediated by mu-receptors and the endogenous opioids, endomorphins-1 and 2.

SEROTONIN THEORY

Recent studies by Lin and Chen (2008) propose that EA may affect the serotonergic descending inhibitory pathway. This pathway is thought to be important in EA analgesia through top-down inhibition of pain signals. Serotonin, a monoamine neurotransmitter, appears to play a part in combination with other neurotransmitters in moderating pain in the central nervous system.

In rodents serotonin antagonists have been used to demonstrate that serotonergic pathways are important in modulating nociceptive signal transmission (Baek *et al.* 2005; Takagi and Yonehara 1998). Tsai, Chen and Lin (1989) found that p-chlorophenylalanine, a serotonin synthesis inhibitor, diminished the analgesic effect of EA.

TISSUE HEALING

Biological electric fields (EF) are generated by the body naturally and are intrinsic to tissue healing. In a resting state the inside of a cell has a negative charge whilst the outside has a positive charge. This difference in charge is called polarization. Depolarisation describes a reversal of this charge due to the movement of ions through ion channels, pumps and protein transporters. Some proteins and enzymes use EF to regulate cell function (Bezanilla 2008). If the depolarization reaches a critical threshold then an "action potential" is triggered. Action potentials form the basis of neuronal communication and thus provide the mechanism behind the propagation of nerve signals and hormone and neurotransmitter release. Neuronal communication can thus be described as electrochemical in nature.

When the body is wounded a steady direct current EF creates an "injury potential". It has been shown that cell migration is guided to the wound edge by this field. By compromising the steady direct current, EF wound healing can be inhibited.

McCaig *et al.* (2005) observed that electrical reactions to injury could persist for a long time across large areas, even beyond the injury site. The authors also noted that when nutritional and metabolic problems arise the electrical properties of certain tissues become abnormal.

Cells are responsive to external electromagnetic fields. Yeast and diatoms (a single cell algae) have been shown to respond to electromagnetic fields (Mehedintu and Berg 1997; Smith *et al.* 1987). These studies suggest that EFs affect the behaviour of cells. Numerous in vitro experiments have demonstrated that EF can affect the adhesion, proliferation, differential, directional migration, as well as division of cells (Meng *et al.* 2011).

The extracellular matrix is an intricate 3-dimensional network of fibrillar proteins, proteoglycans and glycosaminoglycans. This matrix provides an electrochemical network conveying signals in and out of cells. This matrix has been shown to be affected by applying EF and electrical stimulation (ES) (Kotwal and Schmidt 2001).

ES has been found to influence genetic expression. Zhuang *et al.* (1997) found ES increased the gene expression of transforming growth factor-β, (TGF-β), collagen type-I, alkaline phosphatase, bone morphogenetic proteins and the chondrocyte matrix. Meng *et al.* (2008) treated osteoblasts with ES of 200mV/mm for 6 hours and found that osteocalcin and alkaline phosphatase increased by 20% compared to the non-ES control group.

In 1953 Yasuda *et al.* applied continuous electric current to rabbit bone tissue for 3 weeks and found new bone growth in the area where the cathode was positioned. The benefits of ES include formation of fracture callus, faster fracture consolidation, increased resistance to re-fracture, cortical thickening, periosteal and endosteal bone proliferation, reduced incidence of disuse osteoporosis and joint ankyloses (Meng *et al.* 2011). Beck *et al.* (2008) found that treating non-union fractures with capacitive coupling electric fields achieved a success rate of 60-77%.

Although multiple randomised trials exist to demonstrate the various bone healing properties of ES, more definitive trials are needed. Nonetheless, a survey of 450 Canadian orthopaedic surgeons in 2008 by Busse *et al.* found 16% used ES to manage uncomplicated open and closed tibial shaft fractures, whilst almost half (45%) used it in the treatment of complicated tibial shaft fractures.

In 1999 Gardner and colleagues conducted a meta-analysis of the effect of ES on chronic ulcer healing. The results showed a significant reduction in healing time for ulcers treated with ES in comparison to the control. The average rate of wound healing in those treated with ES was 22% per week compared to 9% per week for the control. The authors did not find a significant difference in wound healing rates between treatment protocols: treatment with low intensity direct current, high voltage pulsed current, alternating current and transcutaneous electrical nerve stimulation (TENS) were included.

ES techniques have been found to exert a direct effect on the regeneration of nerves as well as soft tissue and bone. Studies using rat models have shown ES of 2Hz or 20Hz (via implanted or percutaneous electrodes) accelerates axon outgrowth from proximal nerve stumps to distal nerve stumps; in addition, muscle re-innervation was accelerated and facilitation of spinal motor response was reduced (English *et al.* 2007; Geremia *et al.* 2007; Vivo *et al.* 2008). In humans, median nerve regeneration and consequent thenar muscle re-innervation have been accelerated using ES after carpal tunnel release surgery (Gordon *at al.* 2009).

It has been postulated that the milliampere currents

used in TENS are too high to stimulate tissue repair and that microamperes may be more effective (Johnson 2017). A study of percutaneous ES by Lu *et al.* (2009) using milliamperes found that ES of 1mA to 2mA increased nerve stump regeneration whereas ES of 4mA slowed the process. Another study found that microcurrent ES (20Hz, 2µA, 30 minutes) improved functional and sensory recovery, with improvements in sciatic functional index, mean conduction velocity, the number of retrogradely labelled sensory neurones, axon counts and myelin thicknesses (Alrashdan *et al.* 2010).

EFFECTS ON BLOOD FLOW

Kaada (1982) pioneered the use of TENS (burst pattern, frequency of 100Hz) to generate widespread and prolonged cutaneous vasodilation in the management of peripheral ischaemia and symptoms of Raynaud's disease. TENS was found to increase blood plasma serotonin (5-HT), calcitonin gene-related peptide and vasoactive intestinal peptide. Recently it has been suggested that TENS could be of use in preventing venous stasis during surgical treatments; TENS applied to the peroneal nerve increased peak venous velocity and flow volume in the popliteal vein in the limbs of healthy participants (Izumi *et al.* 2010).

MOVES QI AND BLOOD

The application of ES to the human body has been shown in neurological and biochemical research to have multiple sequelae. From a practical working perspective in Chinese medicine I suspect that the main effects of EA are to move qi and Blood. If this assumption is correct, EA is suitable for conditions we would regard as caused by stagnation of qi and Blood i.e. the vast majority of musculoskeletal problems encountered in acupuncture practice.

As a result, in my view, EA is particularly effective for invigorating the circulation in muscles that have become chronically contracted. I believe that this happens firstly by re-establishing the blood flow and secondly by resetting motor signals to the muscles. I suspect that the sustained benefits of EA are less to do with its pain controlling capacity, and more to do with its ability to relax tense muscles and stimulate tissue healing.

REFERENCES

Alrashdan, M.S., Park, J.C., Sung, M.A., Yoo, S.B., Jahng, J.W., Lee, T.H., Kim, S.J., and Lee, J.H. (2010) Thirty minutes of low intensity electrical stimulation promotes nerve regeneration after sciatic nerve crush injury in rat model. *Acta Neurol Belg 110,* 168-79.

Aron, R.K., Boyan, B.D., Ciombor, D.M., Schwartz, Z., and Simon, B.J. (2004) Stimulation of growth factor synthesis by electric and electromagnetic fields. *Clin Orthop Relat Res* 30-37.

Baek, Y.H., Yang, H.I., and Park, D.S. (2005) Analgesic effects of electroacupuncture on inflammatory pain in the rat model of collagen-induced arthritis: mediation by cholinergic and serotonergic receptors. *Brain Research 1057,* 1, 181-185.

Beck, B.R., Matheson, G.O., Bergman, G., Norling, T., Fredericson, M., Hoffman, A.R., and Marcus, R. (2008) Do capacitively coupled electric fields accelerate tibial stress fracture healing? A randomised controlled trial. *American Journal of Sports Medicine 36,* 545-553.

Berg, H., and Zhang, L. (1993) Electrostimulation in cell biology by low-frequency electromagnetic-fields. *Electro and Magnetobiology 12,* 147-163.

Bezanilla, F. (2008) How membrane proteins sense voltage. *Nature Reviews Molecular Cell Biology* 9, 323-332.

Bowsher, D. (1998) Mechanisms of acupuncture; In: Filshie, J., and White, A. (eds) Medical Acupuncture: A western scientific approach. Edinburgh: Churchill Livingstone, 69-82.

Busse, J.W., Morton, E., Lacchetti, C., Guyatt, G.H., and Bhandari, M. (2008) Current management of tibial shaft fracture: A survey of 450 Canadian orthopaedic trauma surgeons. *Acta Orthopaedica 79,* 689-694.

Cameron, M.H. (2012) *Physical Agents in Rehabilitation: from research to practice.* New York: Elsevier Health Sciences.

ELECTROACUPUNCTURE HANDBOOK

Chen, X.H., and Han, J.S. (1992) Analgesia induced by electro-acupuncture of different frequencies is mediated by different types of opioid receptors: another cross-tolerance study. *Behavioural Brain Research 47,* 2, 143-149.

Dharmananda, S. (2002) Electroacupuncture and high frequency electroacupuncture. *Chin Sci Bull 33,* 703-705.

English, A.W., Schwartz, G., Meador, W., and Mulligan, A. (2007) Electrical stimulation promotes peripheral axon regeneration by enhanced neuronal neurotrophin. *Institute for Traditional Medicine.* www.itmonline.org.arts/electro.htm, accessed on 27 July 2015.

Fei, H., Sun, S.L., and Han, J.S. (1988) New evidence supporting differential release of enkephalin and dynorphin by losignalling. *Dev Neurobiol 67,* 158-172.

Ferrier, J., Ross, S.M., Kanehisa, J., and Aubin, J.E. (1986) Osteoclasts and osteoblasts migrate in opposite directions in response to a constant electrical field. *J Cell Physiol 129,* 283-288.

Gardner, S.E., Frantz, R.A., and Schmidt, F.L. (1999) Effect of electrical stimulation on chronic wound healing: meta -analysis. *Wound Repair Regen 7,* 495-503.

Geremia, N.M., Gordon, T., Brushart, T.M., Al-Majed, A.A., and Verge, V.M. (2007) Electrical stimulation promotes sensory neuron regeneration and growth-associated gene expression. *Exp Neurol 205,* 347-359.

Gordon, T., Udina, E., Verge, V.M., and de Chaves, E.I. (2009) Brief electrical stimulation accelerates axon regeneration in the peripheral nervous system and promotes sensory axon regeneration in the central nervous system. *Motor Control 13,* 412-41.

Guo, H.F., Tian, J., Wang, X., Fang, Y., Hou, T., and Han, J. (1996) Brain substrates activated by electroacupuncture of different frequencies (I): comparative study on the expression of oncogene c-fos and genes coding for three opioid peptides. *Molecular Brain Research 43,* 1, 157-166.

Gyer, G., Michael, J., and Tolson, B. (2016) *Dry Needling for Manual Therapists.* London: Singing Dragon.

Han, J.S. (1987) The neurochemical basis of pain relief by acupuncture. A collection of papers 1973-1987. Beijing Medical University, Beijing.

Han, J.S. (1998) The neurochemical basis of pain relief by acupuncture 2. Hubei Science and Technology Press: Wuhan.

Han, Z., Jiang, Y.H., Wan, Y., Wang, Y., Chang, J.K., and Han, J.S. (1999) Endomorphin-1 mediates 2Hz but not 100Hz electro-acupuncture analgesia in rats. *Neuroscience Letters 274,* 2, 75-78.

He, L.F. (1987) Involvement of endogenous opioid peptides in acupuncture analgesia. *Pain 31,*1, 99-121.

Hsieh, C.L., Kuo, C.C., Chen, Y.S., *et al.* (2000) Analgesic effect of electric stimulation of peripheral nerves with different electric frequencies using the formalin test. *American Journal of Chinese Medicine 28,* 2, 291-299.

Huang, C., Li, H.T., Shi, Y.S., Han, J.S., and Wan, Y. (2004) Ketamine potentiates the effect of electroacupuncture on mechanical allodynia in a rat model of neuropathic pain. *Neuroscience Letters 368,* 3, 327-331.

Izumi, M., Ikeuchi, M., Mitani, T., Taniguchi, S., and Tani, T. (2010) Prevention of venous stasis in the lower limb by transcutaneous electrical nerve stimulation. *Eur J Vasc Endovasc Surg 39,* 642-645.

Johnson, I. (2017) Transcutaneous electrical nerve stimulation (TENS) Oxford: Oxford University Press.

Kaada, B. (1982) Vasodilation induced by transcutaneous nerve stimulation in peripheral ischemia (Raynaud's phenomenon and diabetic polyneuropathy). *Eur Heart J 3,* 303-314.

Kotwal, A., and Schmidt, C.E. (2001) Electrical stimulation alters protein absorption and nerve cell interactions with electrically conducting biomaterials. *Biomaterials 22,* 1055-1064.

Leung, L. (2012) Neurophysiological basis of acupuncture-induced analgesia - an updated review. *J. Acupunct. Meridian Stud. 5,*6, 261-270.

Lin, J.G., and Chen, W.L. (2008) Acupuncture analgesia: a review of its mechanisms of actions. *American Journal of Chinese Medicine 36,* 4, 635-645.

Long, D.M. (1974) External electrical stimulation as a treatment of chronic pain. *Minn Med J 57,* 195-198.

Lu, M.C., Tsai, C.C., Chen, S.C., Tsai, F.J., Yao, C.H., and Chen, Y.S. (2009) Use of electrical stimulation at different current levels to promote recovery after peripheral nerve injury in rats. *J Trauma 67,* 10066-10072.

Mayer, D.J., Price, D.D., and Rafii, A. (1977) Antagonism of acupuncture analgesia in man by narcotic antagonist naloxone. *Brain Research 121,* 2, 368-372.

Mayor, D. F. (2007) Electroacupuncture. A practical manual and resource. Edinburgh: Churchill Livingstone.

McCaig, C.D., Rajnicek, A.M., Song, B., and Zhao, M. (2005) Controlling cell behaviour electrically: current views and future potential. *Physiol Rev 85,* 943-978.

Mehedintu, M., and Berg, H. (1997) Proliferation response of yeast saccharomyces cerevisiae on electromagnetic field parameters. *Bioelectrochemistry and Bioenergetics 43,* 67-70.

Meng, S.Y., Rouabhia, M., Shi, G.X., and Zhang, Z. (2008) Heparin dopant increases the electrical stability, cell adhesion and growth of conducting polypyrrole/poly (L,L-lactide) composites. *Journal of Biomedical Materials Research Part A 87A* 332-344.

Meng, S.Y., Rouabhia, M., and Zhang, Z. (2011) Electrical Stimulation in Tissue Regeneration. www.intechopen.com, accessed 25 May 2017.

Melzack, R., and Wall, P.D. (1965) Pain mechanisms: a new theory. *Science.* Nov 19; 150 (3699): 971-9.

Pomeranz, B., Cheng, R., and Law, P. (1977) Acupuncture reduces electrophysiological and behavioural responses to noxious stimuli: pituitary is implicated. *Experimental Neurology 54,* 1, 172-178.

Pomeranz, B., and Chiu, D. (1976) Naloxone blockade of acupuncture analgesia: endorphin implicated. *Life Sciences 19,* 11, 1757-1762.

Shealy, C.N., Mortimer, J.T., and Reswick, J.B. (1967) Electrical inhibition of pain by stimulation of the dorsal columns: preliminary clinical report. *Anesth & Analg 46,* 489-91.

Smith, S.D., McLeod, B.R., Liboff, A.R., and Cooksey, K. (1987) Calcium cyclotron resonance and diatom mobility. *Bioelectromagnetics 8,* 215-227.

Takagi, J., and Yonehara, N. (1998) Serotonin receptor subtypes involved in modulation of electrical acupuncture. *Japanese Journal of Pharmacology 78,* 4, 511-514.

Tsai, H.-Y., Chen, Y.-F., and Lin, J.-G. (1989) Effect of electro-acupuncture analgesia on serotoninergic neurons in rat central nervous system. *Chin Pharmacol J 41,* 123-126.

Vivo, M., Puigdemasa, A., Casals, L., Asensio, E., Udina, E., and Navarro, X. (2008) Immediate electrical stimulation enhances regeneration and reinnervation and modulates spinal plastic changes after sciatic nerve injury and repair. *Exp Neurol 211,* 180-93.

Wall, P.D., and Sweet, W.H. (1967) Temporary abolition of pain in man. *Science 155,* 108-109.

Yasuda, I. (1953) The classic: Fundamental aspects of fracture treatment by Iwao , reprinted from J. Kyoto Med. Soc., 4:395- 406.

Yasuda, I., Noguchi, K., and Sata, T. (1955) Dynamic callus and electrical callus. *J Bone Joint Surg 37a,* 1292-1293.

Yoo, Y.C., Oh, J.H., Kwon, T.D., Lee, Y.K., and Bai, S.J. (2011) Analgesic mechanism of electroacupuncture in an arthritic pain model of rats: a neurotransmitter study. *Yonsei medical Journal 52,* 6, 1016-1021.

Zhuang, H.M., Wang, W., Seldes, R.M., Tahernia, A.D., Fan, H.J., and Brighton, C.T. (1997) Electrical stimulation induces the level of TGF-beta 1 mRNA in osteoblastic cells by a mechanism involving the calcium/calmodulin pathway. *Biochemical and Biophysical Research Communications 237,* 225-229.

Zhao, Z.Q. (2008) Neural mechanism underlying acupuncture analgesia. *Progress in Neurobiology 85,* 4, 355-357.

Electroacupuncture machines

3

On a very simplistic level EA machines involve a battery delivering electricity through a number of paired wires; these pairs are called channels. The machines fall into two basic types: the first are machines that are controlled by knobs and switches and the second are machines controlled by buttons that activate a digital screen. I prefer machines where the intensity function to the channels is controlled by knobs because turning a knob has a more immediate effect than pressing a button when increasing and decreasing the intensity. Knobs are also quicker to turn down or off quickly if the patient suddenly feels extreme discomfort.

When buying an EA machine, consider the size of the machine. If you need a portable machine, smaller would be better. With a larger machine there may be problems fitting it on the couch and so you may need a separate table or stand. Compact machines can simply be placed on the couch next to the patient.

Another important consideration when choosing a machine is its number of channels. Most of the techniques outlined in this book need a maximum of three channels. If, however, you choose to treat two conditions at the same time you may need more channels.

The cost of a machine is usually the best indicator of quality although there are exceptions such as the AWQ series which I used for years and found to be both reliable and economical.

Although EA machines can look very different they are all fundamentally the same, and consist of the following:

- power source (usually a battery or batteries from six to nine volts)

- on/off switch

- output channels - sockets into which pairs of wires with clips are plugged to deliver the electricity to the needles

- intensity controls to adjust the strength of the electrical output delivered to the channels

- frequency controls to adjust how many times per second the electricity changes direction

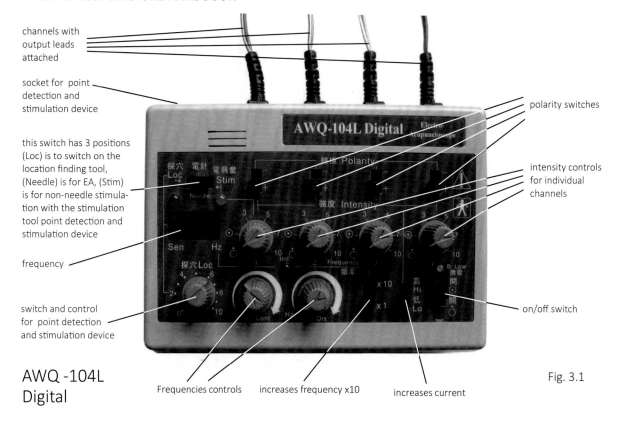

channels with output leads attached

socket for point detection and stimulation device

this switch has 3 positions (Loc) is to switch on the location finding tool, (Needle) is for EA, (Stim) is for non-needle stimulation with the stimulation tool point detection and stimulation device

frequency

switch and control for point detection and stimulation device

polarity switches

intensity controls for individual channels

on/off switch

AWQ -104L Digital

Frequencies controls

increases frequency x10

increases current

Fig. 3.1

- with the AWQ machines there is a second frequency control to create the dense-disperse pattern

- there may be a switch that increases the voltage of the machine by up to a factor of 2 or 3 (so that the device can be used as a TENS machine or for patients who have highly resistant tissue)

- with some machines there is a point detection and stimulation device

- there may also be other controls that further affect the shape of the wave and the phase duration

- Some of the AWQ machines have polarity switches just above the intensity controls. These are the charge balancing switches (only found on machines that are not charge balanced). Their purpose is to make sure that the overall current

moving in one direction during a treatment is exactly the same as the overall current moving in the opposite direction. This avoids the possibility of the corrosive effects of electrolysis at the needles. The switches are used halfway through the treatment to reverse the circuitry thereby equalizing the current in each direction. I do not use the polarity switches myself because treatments are relatively short and therefore any overall difference in cur- rent is likely to be insignificant.

- Some machines have programs of sequences of varying frequencies. As you become more proficient and knowledgeable you may want to experiment with these variables.

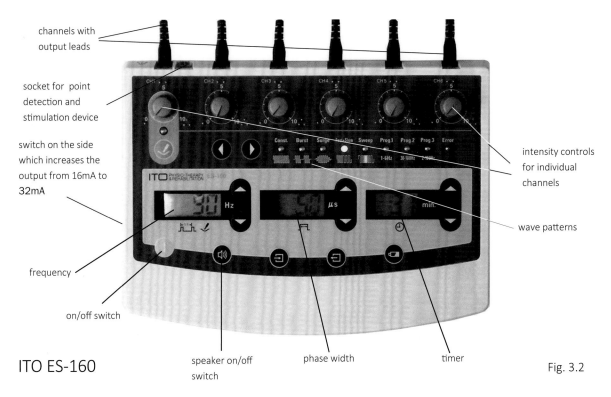

channels with output leads

socket for point detection and stimulation device

switch on the side which increases the output from 16mA to 32mA

intensity controls for individual channels

wave patterns

frequency

on/off switch

speaker on/off switch

phase width

timer

ITO ES-160

Fig. 3.2

AWQ -104L Digital

The AWQ series of EA machines probably goes back to the 1940s. The latest version is the AWQ-105 Pro although I prefer the AWQ-104L Digital (Fig.3.1). Most other makes of machine seem to follow the AWQs' basic layout. The AWQ-104L Digital has an on/off switch, four intensity controls to increase or decrease the electrical output and two knobs to adjust the frequencies which appear on the digital display. It has a switch that can increase the frequency by a factor of 10, a switch to increase voltage from 9 to 27 volts (so that the machine can be used for TENS) and it is also equipped with a point detection and stimulation device on the left hand side.

TO ES-160

Figure 3.2 shows an ITO ES-160. This is a Japanese machine and has roughly the same controls as the AWQ with some extras. It has six output channels with intensity controls and three digital display windows. The first window digitally indicates the frequency, the second window the phase duration (width of one wave) and the third is a timer display indicating the duration of treatment and battery levels, all of which are adjustable using the buttons to the right of the windows. This machine also has a speaker so that you can hear how the different frequencies and wave patterns sound. Higher frequencies create a higher pitch. This is useful when increasing the intensity of DD because the higher frequency tends to be felt more quickly and more strongly than the lower frequency; so the higher pitch alerts you to when the patient might be about to feel a stronger sensation. The speaker also indicates that the machine is working.

17

ELECTROACUPUNCTURE HANDBOOK

There is a choice of set wave-patterns and wave-pattern sequences that can be selected from the buttons along the centre of the machine. There is a switch that increases the overall output of the machine from 16 to 32mA; this is used when more current is required for patients to feel the sensation. It also has a feature for recording the practitioner's own sequences of frequencies. Like the AWQ it has a feature enabling detection and stimulation of points with a probe and a Ryodoraku function for measuring the channel conductivity.

DIGITAL MACHINES

Although I have exclusively used analogue EA machines, I think it is worth mentioning digital machines. I suspect we are moving towards a digital future with EA machines looking like iPhones with a touch screen. One of the advantages of the digital machines is that they are smaller and therefore more portable for the acupuncturist on the move. Being smaller they are also easier to fit on the couch without having to have a trolley or some other device to hold them.

ADJUSTING INTENSITY

Intensity refers to the strength of the electric current delivered to the needles. To ensure the patient remains comfortable and relaxed, it is important not to make the treatment too strong. If the intensity is set correctly the patient will have a pleasant therapeutic experience. If the intensity is too high the muscles contract and possibly go into spasm which is not only painful but can also be dangerous as it can drive the needles deeper into the body. This can be particularly dangerous in the upper back. In addition, putting muscles that are already tight into spasm may, in my opinion, cause further stagnation. Muscle contraction should be totally avoided because the muscle will remain in contraction until the intensity is turned down, causing the patient unnecessary pain.

At lower frequencies (<10Hz) I think that it can be beneficial to allow the treatment to cause gentle muscle contractions: an appropriate setting would be 2/6Hz DD. Even if you do not elicit muscle contrac-   tion it is important to turn the intensity up to a point where the patient can feel it; you then know that the current is definitely flowing through the muscle.

When treating a patient, the intensity controls should be turned up very gradually in slight increments. Turn the control knob up 2 to 3 degrees at a time whilst observing the patient's reaction. Explain to the patient what you are doing and ask them to tell you as soon as they feel tingling, numbness or a full, heavy sensation. For some patients even a tiny adjustment of the control knob can cause a dramatic increase in sensation. Be prepared to turn it down very quickly if the patient feels any discomfort.

If a number of leads are connected to the patient, adjusting the first pair will provide an idea of what level of intensity is comfortable. Sometimes the body gets used to the sensation and the patient is no longer able to feel it; in these circumstances the intensity can be increased again.

Where there are a number of leads in the same area, it is important to note that turning up the intensity in one pair of leads can cause an increase in intensity in another pair of leads. This is because the current flowing between one pair of leads may flow to   another unrelated pair of leads close by. In this situation it may be necessary to decrease the intensity of the first pair before increasing the intensity of the second pair. Always be prepared to turn down the intensity if the patient is feeling uncomfortable and start again.

DURATION OF TREATMENT

EA treatment times can vary from 15 to 30 minutes depending on how chronic the problem is: the more chronic the problem, the longer the treatment required. Although it is often suggested that strong EA treatments can be draining to patients who are deficient (from a TCM perspective), in practice I have not found this to be the case and suspect the idea to be a self-perpetuating myth.

RED AND BLACK LEADS

The red and black leads on EA machines can cause considerable confusion. As mentioned above, because AC current is moving backwards and forwards continuously the charge at the end of each lead is constantly changing from positive to negative - so, generally, it does not matter which way round the leads are placed when using only one pair of leads.

However, when using more than one pair of leads in the same area, one must remember that the electrical flow does not necessarily move exclusively between the two ends of one pair of leads. The current may be attracted to the nearby lead of another pair if its polarity in a particular moment is the opposite to its own.

So if you have two pairs of leads positioned at each end of the same muscle with the intention that the electricity of each pair is to run along the muscle then it is important to position the leads correctly. Both black leads should be positioned together at one end of the muscle and both red leads at the other end. This advice is based on the assumption that when both black leads are positive, both red leads are negative and vice versa at any given moment.

Of course in practice it is not always possible to arrange the leads in this way because of the close proximity of a number of different leads, but it is worth bearing in mind when there is a choice.

STORING THE LEADS

It is common practice to store the EA leads by winding them around the machine. The winding and unwinding of the leads can take a considerable time and they often get tangled in the process. A way of avoiding this is to get a small stainless steel tray that is about the same size as the machine (Fig. 3. 3) from a kitchen shop or Chinese medical supplier. The tray should have shallow sides and a lip around the edge. Instead of winding the leads round the machine you can clip them to the edge of the tray and leave them dangling down (Fig. 3. 4). Using this method you will save time and avoid the frustration of tangled leads.

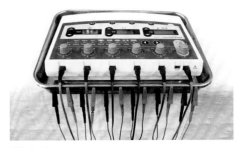

Fig 3. 3

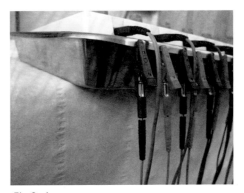

Fig 3. 4

Precautions and contraindications

4

Common sense should be the guiding principle when it comes to safety, and EA treatment should generally adhere to the safety precautions observed during any acupuncture treatment. Below are listed some additional considerations:

- Ensure all intensity controls are at zero before switching on the machine; otherwise you may give the patient an unpleasant shock. Also turn down the intensity controls before switching the machine off. In the past, some machines created a sudden surge in electricity when the machine was switched off. In any case, it is good practice to turn down the intensity controls at the end of each session in preparation for the next.

- Always turn the intensity control up very slowly, and be ready to turn it down quickly if the muscles start to contract.

- If two pairs of EA needles are in close proximity the patient may report that the sensation at the first pair of needles becomes more intense when you turn up the second pair. In this situation you need to reduce the intensity of the first pair before turning up the second pair.

- Make sure that the leads are supported rather than allowing the full weight of the leads to pull on the needles. Not only can the leads fall out easily, but the tugging of the leads can cause the needles to be painful.

- Be aware that any involuntary contraction of the muscles caused by the intensity setting being too high can cause the needles to be driven deeper into the body. Be particularly cautious of this when treating the upper back because of the close proximity of the lungs.

- Attach the clips at the base of the needles so that if the muscle contracts, the needles are less likely to be drawn deeper into the body. Also, by attaching the clips at the base of the needles they are less likely to be pulled out by the leads.

- Muscles can go into involuntary contraction if the patient tries to move the muscles that are being treated with EA. The reason for this is that their own electrical motor signals combine with the EA signal causing a greater contraction. So it is important to encourage the patient to remain still and relaxed during a treatment.

- Do not place electrodes across the carotid sinus as this can cause a sudden drop in blood pressure.

- Avoid EA around the eyes.

- Do not use EA on patients with pacemakers.

- Avoid the cardiac region Ren-12 to SP-21 on the left side of the body.

- Avoid crossing the chest or upper back.

- Do not use EA on recent fractures as it may cause muscle contraction and misalign the bone.

- Never use a TENS machine for EA as it is too strong.

- EA can be used during pregnancy, but avoid EA on MA points that are contraindicated in pregnancy and points in the lumbar region unless you are trying to induce the baby.

- EA appears not to suit everyone, and can temporarily exacerbate pain in about one in ten patients. If this exacerbation is followed by relief then it is generally worth continuing with the treatment, but if EA exacerbates the problem for a number of days without improvement then manual acupuncture should be resumed.

For a more extensive list of precautions and contraindications see *Electroacupuncture* by David Mayor.

ATTACHING THE EA CLIPS SAFELY TO THE NEEDLES

The EA clips should be positioned on the shaft of the needle and in contact with the skin surface rather than on the handle of the needle; this minimizes any leverage that would be caused by placing the clips on the handle of the needle (Fig. 4. 1). Clearly acupuncture needles are not structurally designed for EA. By positioning the clips strategically, it is possible to minimise this problem.

Positioning the clips is not so much of a problem when the needles are relatively perpendicular; the

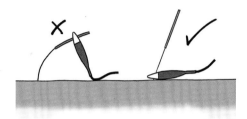

Fig. 4. 1

real problem arises when the needles are horizontal, sticking out from the side of the body. It is important to avoid using longer needles than you need to, further minimising any unnecessary leverage. If the patient is in a sitting position having a shoulder treatment you can use 15mm needles on TH-14 and LI-15; if you insert them up to the hilt and attach the clips to the handle next to the skin they are unlikely to fall out. Similarly, if you are treating carpal tunnel syndrome using SI-5 and LI-5 you can use 15mm needles in the same way. This short needle approach

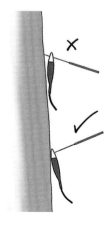

Fig. 4. 2

is mainly used when you are not treating the muscles directly e.g. carpal tunnel syndrome and plantar fasciitis. The important consideration with these conditions is to penetrate just below the epidermis, so that the electricity is introduced to the more moist conductive layer of the interior of the body. Obviously deeper needling is necessary when you are treating the muscles themselves.

Another way to reduce the possibility of needles coming out when they are inserted horizontally is to place the needles at an angle so that the end of the handle is higher than the point of insertion (Fig. 4. 2).

It is also important to support the leads by draping them along the body or couch. You can also place cotton wool balls under a needle and clip if they need further support. Some people use sticky tape to support the needles.

EXTREME CAUTION WHEN TREATING THE UPPER BACK

It is of course of paramount importance to be cautious when needling the upper back with manual acupuncture, but with EA we need to be even more vigilant. The reason for this is that when using EA the needles can move rhythmically at low frequencies with the possible consequence of driving the needles deeper into the back resulting in a possible pneumothorax.

When treating points in the upper back away from the spine I would recommend you use needles no longer than 15mm with the clip attached to the shaft rather than the handle; this means the depth of penetration does not exceed 10mm (Fig. 4. 3). With some very thin patients even this may be too deep and, conversely, with obese people or patients with well developed back muscles deeper needling with longer needles may be necessary. My point here is that one should proceed with caution. With the EA clip placed on the shaft of the needle you have complete control of needle depth and no possibility of the needles being driven further into the body. If you are considering bilateral treatment of the upper back with EA and do not feel confident, limit the treatment to one side per session: a person can survive a unilateral pneumothorax but a bilateral pneumothorax is potentially fatal. Fortunately the problems we treat in the upper back are more commonly one-sided.

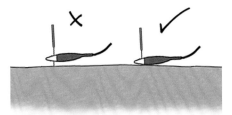

Fig. 4. 3

Treatment principles

5

The following chapters describe a number of treatment protocols for various musculo-skeletal problems. The principles of treatment fall into three main categories.

1. STIMULATING MUSCLES

Stimulation along the muscle fibres in order to re-establish normal muscle function where there has been long term chronic contraction or injury. Initially I would use low frequencies (3Hz/6Hz DD) without inducing obvious muscle contraction and see if this works; then progress to eliciting gentle rhythmic muscle contractions and see if this is more or less effective. Some patients need very little stimulation to achieve good results; others need stronger stimulation.

2. STIMULATING JOINTS, CARTILAGE, VERTEBRAL DISCS & TENDONS

Treating joints, cartilage, vertebral discs and tendons by stimulating the healing properties of the body by passing electricity around or through the area.

3. DISRUPTING NERVE SIGNALS TO REDUCE PAIN

Disruption of nerve signals to reduce pain. This can be achieved by applying EA along the spine at the spinal segment related to specific conditions such as sciatica. This may of course have the simultaneous effect of releasing any tight vertebral muscles that are trapping the spinal nerves which might have caused the pain in the first place. EA can also be applied across tendon insertions to reduce pain when treating conditions like tennis elbow. I suspect that any reduction in pain from EA is due more to the healing effects of EA on the tissues being treated than the pain relieving properties of electricity.

USING MULTIPLE MODALITIES

With some conditions we can use 2 or 3 of these approaches in one treatment simultaneously e.g. for tennis elbow, treating both the muscle and the insertion of the tendon. It is not necessary to stick rigidly to the frameworks described; once the general principles have been grasped they can be applied to all sorts of conditions.

TREATING THE UNDERLYING CONSTITUTION

I cannot emphasise enough the importance of also treating the underlying constitutional causes from a Chinese medical perspective. This may be the difference between success and failure. Localized EA may well be dramatic and effective in the short term but will only have lasting effects when the underlying constitutional causes are addressed. Sustained benefits will also only be realized by addressing other lifestyle issues like diet, posture and exercise. Although remedial exercises are beyond the remit of this book I have included exercises for neck and back problems which I believe are essential for a successful outcome.

WHEN TO USE EA

EA can be used for all the conditions described in this book, particularly when the condition is chronic and/or degenerative. EA can make an enormous difference to these conditions in ways that manual acupuncture cannot. Numerous patients will testify to the efficacy of EA over manual acupuncture. Once you become familiar with the techniques and their effectiveness, it is unlikely that you will go back to just using manual acupuncture.

MANUAL STIMULATION

Generally speaking, manual stimulation of the needles to which EA is being applied is unnecessary, particularly when you are using a lot of needles. In this situation it is only necessary to stimulate the constitutional and distal points manually.

THREADING NEEDLE TECHNIQUE

Perpendicular needling is effective for most of the procedures outlined in this book unless otherwise stated. However, when a technique is not working it is worth trying EA with a threading technique.

Instead of inserting the needles perpendicular to the skin you insert them at an angle following the direction of the muscle fibres. If you have two needles at each end of a particular muscle you direct them so that the needles are pointing towards each other. When treating a tendon you thread the needles horizontally either side of the tendon. Using this method you are exposing more of the tissue to the needle and the electrical stimulation.

CHOICE OF POINTS

Although many of the points used for electroacupuncture in this system are traditional acupuncture points, they are primarily chosen because they are located in the correct position to treat the joints, muscles and tendons. The supplementary channel points are of course used for their traditional functions.

WHAT FREQUENCY SHALL I USE?

For the purpose of this book I have decided to define frequencies in the following way:

- LOW FREQUENCY 1 to 6Hz

- MEDIUM FREQUENCY 20 to 60Hz

- HIGH FREQUENCY 100Hz and above

A vast range of frequencies is employed in electrotherapy, from 1Hz to frequencies as high as 4000Hz (used by physiotherapists for interferential therapy). Transcutaneous electrical nerve stimulation (TENS) machines use frequencies between 60 and 130Hz. The parameters of frequency used for EA tend to be between 1 and 100Hz, although my ITO ES-160 can deliver frequencies of 500Hz. For many years I was under the impression that low frequencies (i.e. from 1 to 10Hz) stimulate motor neurons and high frequencies (i.e. 80 to 100Hz) affect sensory neurons (Walsh and Berry 2010). This would suggest that low frequencies are more effective for treating muscular dysfunction and high frequencies are more effective for treating sensory problems such as pain.

For the first 15 years my machine was set on 30/90Hz DD and I seemed to get perfectly good results. After further research I followed the protocol of using low frequencies to treat the motor nerves and high frequencies to treat the sensory nerves. For a period I would typically first apply 2/6Hz DD along the muscle fibres (to affect the motor neurons) and then 100Hz DD across a tendon insertion (to affect the sensory neurons). This didn't particularly improve the outcome. In practice I have found both low frequencies (2/6Hz DD) and relatively high frequencies (33/100Hz DD) effective for treating musculoskeletal problems. I have met practitioners who use very low frequencies and very high frequencies effectively. I suspect that the reason for EA being considerably more effective than MA for specific conditions is the use of electricity per se rather than specific frequencies being used. Hopefully further research will resolve this question conclusively.

Despite the fact that relatively high frequencies (33/100Hz DD) may be effective for treating muscles, there are two reasons why I currently use low frequencies (2/6Hz DD). The first is that when increasing the intensity using low frequencies, the stimulation comes on relatively slowly and so the patient does not feel the sudden unpleasant contraction of a muscle which may occur at higher frequencies. The second reason is that the slow pulsing contraction and relaxation of the muscle at low frequencies is more therapeutic in terms of normalising muscle function. This does not mean of course that you have to have any visible contraction and relaxation to have a therapeutic effect.

Medium frequencies (i.e. 6/20Hz DD) I tend to think of as having a healing effect on joints and tendons; much higher frequencies (i.e. 100/300Hz DD) I tend to use for penetrating old scar tissue, the nodules of Dupuytren's contracture or bony joints. The thinking here is that higher frequencies have a more penetrating effect, but I have not come across any evidence to support this notion.

On a practical note, in terms of record keeping, I think that it is really important to record what frequencies you use: some frequencies seem to benefit some patients more than others; it is therefore vital to keep a record so that you can repeat a treatment that has been effective. It is also a way of accumulating a body of knowledge both for your own practice and for the wider acupuncture community.

RESEARCH ON FREQUENCY

Jisheng Han's Beijing group (Han 1987; Han 1998) demonstrated that different frequencies affected different brain nuclei. They discovered that 2Hz EA mediated the spinal cord μ and δ opioid receptors, 100Hz affected κ receptors and 2/15Hz DD affected all three.

Research revealed 2Hz EA applied to rats stimulated the production of met-enkephalin. It has also been discovered that 2Hz EA at the spinal level influences endorphin and endomorphin-1. In the brain, enkephalin synthesis within the hypothalamic arcuate nucleus is also affected by low frequency EA (Han 1987; Han 1998). 15Hz EA can affect spinal neurotransmitters including dynorphin, substance P and angiotensin II. In the spinal cord dynorphin has been released using 100Hz.

Mayor (2007) observed that low frequency has more general analgesic effect whereas high frequency has a more localized analgesic effect.

IS EA SUITABLE FOR TRADITIONAL ACUPUNCTURE?

In my experience EA is not more effective than MA in stimulating the meridians using the TCM model; in fact it can have an adverse effect. I treated a menopausal woman who had had a total hysterectomy including the ovaries and was experiencing extreme hot flushes day and night. The treatment with MA was going very well with considerable reduction in her flushes. I thought that I might be able to enhance the treatment by applying EA to Ren Mai (Lu-7 to Ki-6). The hot flushes immediately came back with a vengeance. I have also tonified back shu points with EA with no noticeable advantage over MA. I have tried treating migraine by applying EA from Gb-20 to Gb-43, again with no noticeable advantages over MA. That is not to say that EA may not be successfully used to treat the meridian systems in the future, but at present I only use EA to treat musculoskeletal problems.

PALPATION AS DIAGNOSIS

Most of the techniques outlined in this book rely on a diagnosis based on palpation in order to find points to treat. Sometimes muscles may appear or feel tight, but have no ashi points. In these situations choose points at either side of a tight area in the muscle so that when applying EA the electricity flows along the muscle in order to release the chronic contraction.

THIS BOOK

The following chapters describe how to treat specific musculoskeletal problems with EA. As this book is primarily aimed at traditional acupuncturists I have not discussed these problems from a Chinese medical perspective in any depth as they are well documented elsewhere. I have however briefly described these conditions from a western point of view, in addition to providing my own insights and ideas. The following chapters each include a concise description of the relevant anatomical structures of the body in support of the various treatment approaches.

Han, J.S. (1987) The neurochemical basis of pain relief by acupuncture. A collection of papers 1973-1987. Beijing Medical University, Beijing.

Han, J.S. (1998) The neurochemical basis of pain relief by acupuncture 2. Hubei Science and Technology Press, Wuhan.

Mayor, D. F. (2007) Electroacupuncture. A practical manual and resource. Edinburgh: Churchill Livingstone.

Walsh, S., and Berry, K. (2010) Electroacupuncture and TENS: Putting theory into practice. *Journal of Chinese Medicine 92*.

Neck pain

6

Neck pain (or cervicalgia) has become a very common problem with our increasingly sedentary lifestyle. In particular, sitting in front of computers in an unnaturally rigid position inevitably leads to the musculature of the neck, shoulders and back becoming tight. Constantly looking down at mobile phones exacerbates the problem. As the head moves forward from the vertical position the load on the neck muscles increases considerably. As the muscles tighten, the blood supply becomes restricted and pain and stiffness can arise. If the contraction of the muscles persists the intervertebral nerves in the neck can become trapped eventually giving rise to nerve pain and tingling down the arms. If the problem continues over a period of time, disc herniation can occur and degenerative conditions like spondylosis arise.

Another cause of neck problems is that many of the muscles supporting the arms attach to the neck and upper back adding more load on the neck. This load is increased by lifting heavy objects. Moreover, the neck muscles are a place where people can habitually hold tension and stress. So it is not surprising to find

that this area is particularly vulnerable. Chronically tight, stiff necks can also give rise to chronic headaches. Poor posture can exacerbate any problems by adding an extra load to the muscles. Once a chronic neck problem has become established it is difficult to remedy without addressing all these issues.

Many musculoskeletal problems can start with trauma. With neck problems that could of course be whiplash. Another contributory factor is that neck problems, like all musculoskeletal problems, can occur against a background of autoimmune disorders like polymyalgia rheumatica, rheumatoid arthritis and multiple sclerosis. Fibromyalgia is also often categorized with these disorders, though it has yet to be officially classified as an autoimmune disorder.

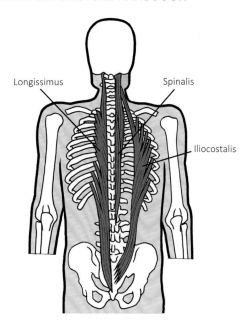

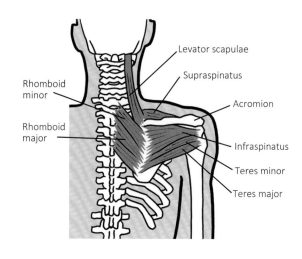

Erector spinae muscles

UNDERLYING STRUCTURES

When treating a neck problem from a musculo-skeletal perspective it is important to view the problem within the context of the whole back. The back muscles involved are the erector spinae muscles which include the iliocostalis, longissimus and spinalis. The iliocostalis and longissimus run from the neck to the sacrum. The spinalis muscle runs from the neck to the beginning of the lumbar spine. Tightness in these muscles is a common cause of neck pain. The erector spinae muscles roughly coincide with the outer Bladder channel, inner Bladder channel and huatuojiaji points from a TCM channel perspective.

Although the pain may be experienced in the neck itself the cause may be tight spinae erector muscles in the mid or lower back. It is not unusual to find tight ashi points in the lower and mid back (and even in the quadratus lumborum) which are related to neck problems. Another muscle that is commonly implicated in neck pain is the levator scapulae. It originates at the transverse processes of the atlas and axis, as well as at the posterior tubercles of the 3rd and 4th cervical vertebrae, and inserts at the superior medial border of the scapula. It is important to establish the extent of any muscular tension running through the back by palpating thoroughly.

Other muscles that affect the neck are the scalenes, splenius, sternocleidomastoids and the trapezius. In practice I have found them to be far less important in the majority of neck problems than the erector spinae and levator scapulae muscles. Once a neck problem is well established, other muscles may be drawn into the problem like the rhomboids, teres major or minor. These muscles can usually be treated with MA alone, but occasionally EA is needed.

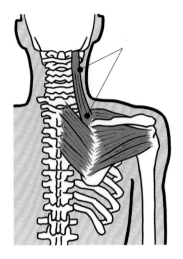
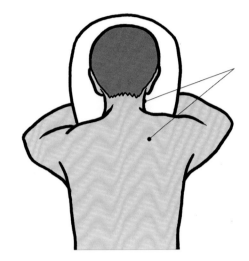

Levator scapulae

In this example the primary points of tenderness are at the superior and inferior insertions of the levator scapulae. They can be found on the lateral side of the neck and on the superior medial border of the scapula at SI-13. There may be other ashi points on the rhomboids, trapezius, teres major or minor that need treating with MA.

1 With the patient in a prone position and their head preferably in a head support, palpate the lateral and posterior aspects of the neck as well as the shoulder and whole back from the base of the neck to the sacrum along the iliocostalis and longissimus. Then palpate the spinalis muscles from the base of the neck to the lower thoracic region. Also check for sore points in the infraspinatus, rhomboids, supraspinatus, teres major and minor.

If the primary problem is in the levator scapulae muscle the main points of tenderness will be around SI-13 at the inferior insertion of the muscle and at the superior insertion on the side of the neck.

2 Needle the tender point on the side of the neck and also the tender point around SI-13. Attach EA clips.

3 Needle any other ashi points in the muscles over the scapula and back using MA.

4 Add musculoskeletal channel points with MA: SI-3, SI-6, Bl-10, Bl-60, Bl-63, GB-20, GB-39, Luozhen (M-UE-24).

5 Add constitutional points with MA.

6 Turn on the EA machine, set the frequency to 6/2Hz DD and carefully turn up the intensity to a point where the patient feels a comfortable tingling or pulsing sensation. Treat with EA for 10 to 20 minutes.

CAUTION

As with all points used in the upper back the same precautions outlined in chapter 4 should be adopted.

31

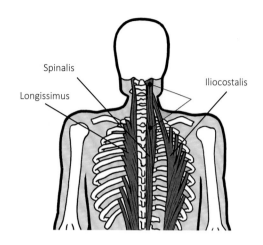

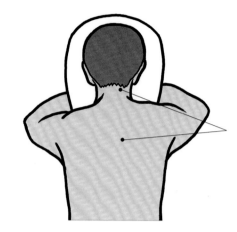

Spinalis

In this presentation neck pain is caused by tension in the spinalis muscle which is close to the spine in the cervical and upper thoracic areas running along the huatuojiaji points.

1 With the patient in a prone position and their head preferably in a head support, palpate the lateral and posterior aspects of the neck as well as the shoulder and whole back along the iliocostalis, longissimus and spinalis muscles. Also check for sore points in the infraspinatus, rhomboids, supraspinatus, teres major and minor. If the primary problem is in the spinalis muscle you will find tender points in the neck and upper back on one or both sides close to the spine. The spinalis muscle actually consists of three muscles: the spinalis capitis, spinalis cervicis and spinalis thoracis; but for practical purposes can be considered one muscle running close to the spine along the huatuojiaji points. Often the points of tenderness in the upper back are around T4 to T6 where the back curves forward. The main point of tenderness in the neck is usually around BI-10 at the superior end of the spinalis muscle. As with all points used in the upper back the same precautions outlined in chapter 4 should be adopted.

2 Insert a needle in a tender point on the neck inferior to the occipital bone closer to BI-10 than GB-20 (if there are no tender points in the neck use BI-10) and another needle in the spinalis muscle lateral to the spine in the mid upper back. Needles can also be placed between these two points particularly if the points are sore or tight, using MA. If it is a considerable distance between the neck and back points, more needles can be added at alternate huatuojiaji points or every three vertebrae. Usually this is unnecessary but worth considering where there is an intractable problem. Attach EA clips to the neck point and thoracic point.

3 Needle any other ashi points in the muscles over the scapula and back using MA.

4 Add musculoskeletal channel points with MA: SI-3, SI-6, BI-10, BI-60, BI-63, GB-20, GB-39 and constitutional points.

5 Turn on the EA machine, set the frequency to 6/2Hz DD and carefully turn up the intensity to a point where the patient feels a comfortable tingling or pulsing sensation. Treat with EA for 10 to 20 minutes.

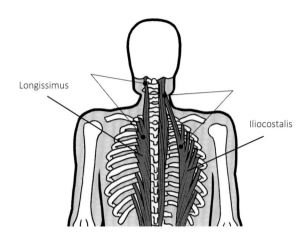

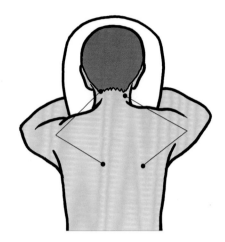

Iliocostalis & longissimus

In this presentation neck pain is arising from either the iliocostalis or longissimus muscles. They are presented together here to compare their locations but rarely occur together in practice.

1 With the patient in a prone position and their head preferably in a head support, palpate the lateral and posterior aspects of the neck as well as the shoulder and whole back along the iliocostalis, longissimus and spinalis muscles. Also check for sore points in the infraspinatus, rhomboids, supraspinatus, teres major and minor.

If the primary problem is in the iliocostalis or longissimus muscles you will not only find ashi points in the neck but also in the iliocostalis and longissimus muscles further down the back. Often the points of tenderness in the upper back are where the upper back starts to curve forward at T4 to T6 which is where the muscles are under maximum stress. The main points of tenderness in the neck will be around Bl-10 and GB-20.

2 Insert a needle in a tender point on the neck inferior to the occipital bone between Bl-10 and GB-20; if there are no tender points in the neck use Bl-10. Insert another needle in a tender point along the iliocostalis or longissimus muscle. Needles can also be placed between these two points, particularly if the points are sore or tight, using MA. Usually this is unnecessary but worth considering with persistent problems. Attach EA clips to the neck point and thoracic point.

3 Needle any other ashi points in the muscles over the scapula and back using MA.

4 Add musculoskeletal channel points with MA: SI-3, SI-6, Bl-10, Bl-60, Bl-63, GB-20, GB-39, Luozhen (M-UE-24).

5 Add constitutional points with MA.

6 Turn on the EA machine, set the frequency to 6/2Hz DD and carefully turn up the intensity to a point where the patient feels a comfortable tingling or pulsing sensation. Treat with EA for 10 to 20 minutes.

CAUTION

As with all points used in the upper back the same precautions outlined on page 23 should be adopted.

NECK EXERCISES

Chronic neck problems can be difficult to treat as discussed at the beginning of this chapter. It is therefore important to give your patient exercises and other advice to break the cycle of tension.

1. If the patient is habitually holding their shoulders high, help them to realise this and get them into the habit of constantly dropping their shoulders during the day. You can suggest triggers like dropping their shoulders when the phone rings or when having to stop at red traffic lights. Many everyday situations can be used as triggers. If they always hold their phone in their right hand and the problem is on the right hand side of the neck, suggest they answer the phone with the other hand while consciously relaxing their right shoulder.

2. If they have poor posture this will lead to extra strain on the neck, so encouraging them to adopt a better posture can be very helpful.

3. For patients with very poor posture, periods lying on the floor on their backs with their head supported can help improve posture by gently opening and straightening up the back.

4. Below are three exercises I recommend.

SHOULDER ROLLING

This exercise is best performed in a standing position. Commence with the arms hanging down at your sides. Then slowly raise the shoulders towards the ears, still with the arms hanging down, and then roll them forward in a circular movement, moving down to their lowest position and consciously letting go of the muscles. Next, lift the shoulders drawing them back in an arc, creating a continuous circular movement. Then repeat the movement in reverse. The emphasis here is on lowering, loosening and relaxing the shoulder muscles.

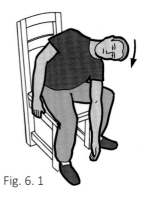

Fig. 6. 1

SEATED STRETCH

This is best performed in a chair with the feet placed at 90° to one another. When stretching the right side of the neck, gently bend over to the left knee, sliding the left arm down the inside of the left leg, tilting the left ear towards the left knee (Fig. 6. 1). This gives an excellent stretch to the levator scapulae and the trapezius and is much more effective than tilting the neck laterally in an upright sitting position which can easily sprain the neck.

NECK TWIST

This is a simple exercise which involves just slowly turning the head from left to right which stretches and loosens the deep intervertebral muscles.

BALL MASSAGE

This self-massage is performed with a hard rubber ball: lacrosse balls are very good; tennis balls and prickly massage balls are too soft. Standing with their back to the wall the patient places the ball between their upper back and the wall (Fig. 6. 2) and then massages their upper back and neck by bending their knees and rolling the ball up and down on their upper back/neck. The ball can also be moved from side to side. A gentle massage twice a day for 5 minutes can really free up very hard knotty muscles.

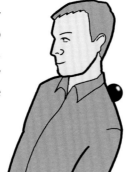

Fig. 6. 2

CASE STUDY

This 67 year old woman presented with neck and upper back pain particularly between the shoulder blades. She works as a podiatrist and so has spent much of her working life leaning forward. She has a history of breast cancer, breast lumps, constipation, digestive problems, glandular fever, lumbar disc problems, menopausal flushes and migraines. She complained of not having the strength to hold her head up. From a TCM perspective I believe her original primary problem to be Spleen qi deficiency with Liver qi stagnation and more recently some Kidney yin deficiency.

EXAMINATION

On palpation much of the upper back and neck was tender and sore, particularly along the iliocostalis, levator scapulae, longissimus and trapezius muscles.

TREATMENT

Initial treatment was directed at relieving the tightness and tension in the iliocostalis, levator scapulae, longissimus and trapezius muscles, with and without EA, and strengthening Spleen and Kidney. Although this improved the situation, she still complained of pain between the shoulder blades along the spinalis muscles. The following treatment specifically focused on the spinalis muscles.

1. Applied EA along the spinalis muscles from Bl-10 to the huatuojiaji points at T8 on either side of the spine.
2. Added ashi points along the spinalis muscles using the huatuojiaji points at the level of C7, T2 and T5 with MA.
3. Added musculoskeletal points with MA: SI-3, SI-6, GB-39, Bl-63, Bl-65.
4. Added constitutional points with MA: Bl-20, Bl-23, Du-20, Du-6, Du-4, Du-3, Ki-6, Sp-3.

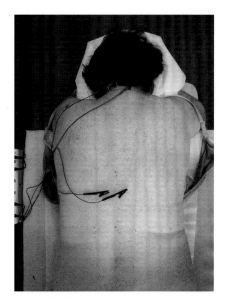

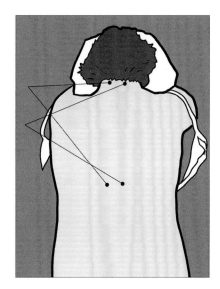

OUTCOME

Treating the spinalis muscles dramatically improved the situation. With monthly treatments she continued to work until her pending retirement without having to lie on the floor in the middle of the day to relieve the pain.

CASE STUDY

This 69 year old female presented with a stiff neck that she had had for 18 months. Her neck was so stiff she could hardly move it at all. Her accompanying symptoms were stiff painful knees that were worse in damp weather and a tendency to overheat especially at night. The pulses were so overwhelmingly wiry that most of the points I used were to move Liver qi. I suspect that the extreme rigidity of the neck had deep-seated emotional causes. Underlying the extreme Liver qi stagnation was Spleen qi deficiency.

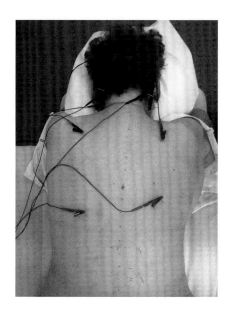

EXAMINATION

Palpation revealed that there was soreness at the superior and inferior insertions of the levator scapulae. Also the iliocostalis muscles on both sides were sore and tight.

TREATMENT

1. Applied EA at the superior and inferior insertions of the levator scapulae on both sides.

2. Applied EA from GB-20 to points midway down the back on the iliocostalis on both sides.

3. Added musculoskeletal points with MA: SI-3, Bl-65 for the neck.

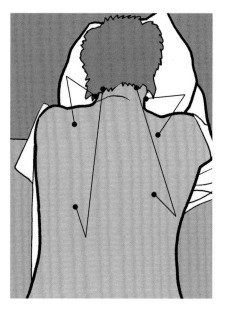

4. Added constitutional points with MA: Du-8, Bl-18, TH-6, LI-4, Liv-3, GB-39.

Once the pulses were less wiry, I started addressing the underlying Spleen deficiency and included points to benefit the joints directly: Bl-20, Du-6, St-34, Sp-5, Sp-9, Ren-12.

OUTCOME

She responded well from the first treatment and progressed steadily. Her neck made a total recovery and her knees were considerably less stiff.

syndrome with generalised stiffness in her joints exacerbated by cold and damp.

EXAMINATION

It is not unusual to see chronic neck pain developing into lower back pain over a period of time as the tight neck muscles start to pull on the lower back muscles. In terms of the muscles affected in the neck there was tightness and soreness in the levator scapulae and the spinalis muscle from C7 to T4. In the lumbar region there was tightness in the longissimus muscle from T12 to L5 and also in the superior and inferior borders of the quadratus lumborum. All the symptoms were on the left side.

TREATMENT

1. Applied EA along the spinalis from C7 to T4 on the left.

2. Applied EA from the insertion of the levator scapulae muscle in the neck to the insertion on the upper medial border of the scapula at SI-13 on the left side.

3. Applied EA along the longissimus muscle from T12 to L5 on the left side.

4. Applied EA from the superior to the inferior borders of the quadratus lumborum on the left side.

5. Added musculoskeletal points with MA: SI-3, GB-34, GB-39, Bl-40, Bl-65 on the left side.

6. Added constitutional points with MA: B-20, Bl-23, Du-6, Du-4 with moxa, Du-3 with moxa, Ki-7, Sp-5, St-41.

OUTCOME

After 8 treatments the pain in the neck and lumbar region were resolved. The patient initially came for 4 weeks weekly and then fortnightly. For homework I suggested the back exercises outlined in this book.

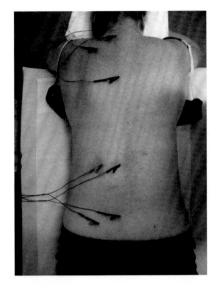

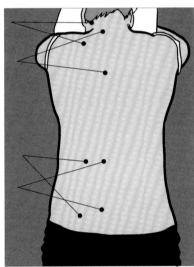

CASE STUDY

This 41 year old woman presented with neck problems and lower back problems on the left side. The symptoms of pain and stiffness were accompanied by tingling and burning down the left arm and leg. The problem was probably due to her job as a lorry driver and a road traffic accident 15 years previously. The underlying constitutional factors are some Spleen qi deficiency and yang deficiency giving rise to Damp bi

Shoulder

7

Bursitis, frozen shoulder, osteoarthritis & rheumatoid arthritis

Frozen shoulder (also known as adhesive capsulitis) is a disorder of unclear cause in which the shoulder capsule and the connective tissue surrounding the glenohumeral joint become inflamed and stiff. Frozen shoulder can be very painful and debilitating and is often worse at night and in cold weather. Certain movements or jolting of the shoulder can provoke episodes of pain and cramping. Frozen shoulder can be caused by trauma and is thought to have an autoimmune component but can also occur for no specific known reason. Movement of the shoulder can be severely restricted with progressive loss of both active and passive range of movement. The condition usually has three stages:

1. The 'freezing' or painful stage, which may last from six weeks to nine months, is a period where there is a gradual onset of pain and stiffness.
2. The 'frozen' or adhesive stage is characterised by a reduction of pain and increase in stiffness and immobility of the shoulder. This can last from four to nine months.
3. The 'thawing' stage, when the stiffness starts to abate, and normal movement is restored. This period can last from 5 to 26 months.

Osteoarthritis commences with localised degeneration of a joint through wear and tear progressing to a painful inflammatory state - usually affecting only one joint. Rheumatoid arthritis, on the other hand, is a systemic autoimmune disease that may affect a number of joints throughout the body. EA is very effective for both these conditions.

Of all the techniques outlined in this book the treatment of frozen shoulder is the least effective. In my experience, EA can be helpful in reducing pain and increasing movement but further progress is often limited. However, treatment of osteo or rheumatoid arthritis of the shoulder with these techniques can be very effective. EA seems to be more effective in treating muscles than connective tissue; this may be because muscles have a better blood supply and so can recover more easily than tendons and other connective tissue.

UNDERLYING STRUCTURES

The shoulder joint is supported by deep and superficial muscles. The deeper muscles that attach to the head of the humerus forming the rotator cuff are the infraspinatus, supraspinatus, teres minor and subscapularis. These muscles are important in stabilising the glenohumeral joint (Figs 7. 1 and 7. 2).

On the anterior aspect of the shoulder (Fig 7. 3) the pectoralis major and minor (not illustrated) attach to the anterior head of the humerus. The latissimus dorsi muscle attaches to the medial side of the humerus just below the humeral head (not illustrated). Covering the shoulder is the deltoid whose origins are in the acromion process, clavicle and spine of the scapula and attaches to the deltoid tuberosity halfway down the lateral surface of the humerus.

Other muscles that can have an influence on the shoulder are the levator scapulae, the rhomboids and teres major (Fig 7. 1).

Any tightness in any of the shoulder muscles can restrict mobility of the joint and exacerbate the frozen shoulder. This muscular restriction can also increase any underlying inflammation from osteo- or rheumatoid arthritis.

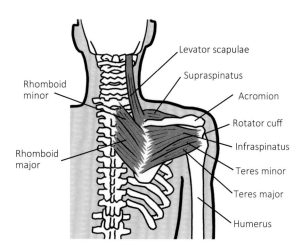

Fig 7. 1   VIEW FROM POSTERIOR

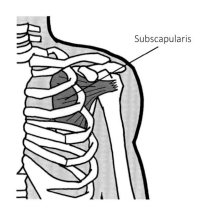

Fig 7. 2   VIEW FROM ANTERIOR

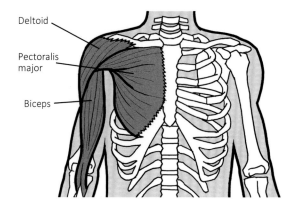

Fig 7. 3   VIEW FROM ANTERIOR

40

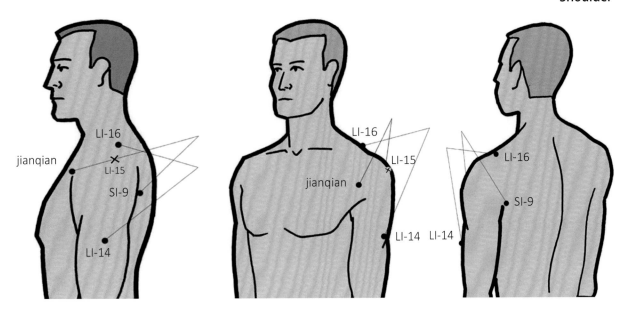

Basic shoulder treatment

From an EA point of view it is not necessary to differentiate between frozen shoulder and osteo or rheumatoid arthritis of the shoulder as the local treatment is the same for all three.

Before commencing any EA of the shoulder joint, palpate the subscapularis muscle (ideally with the patient lying on their back with their arm raised above their head). Check for any ashi points and treat these with MA. Treating the subscapularis can make a significant difference in a handful of cases.

Shoulder problems are best treated with the patient in a sitting position; this gives full access to the posterior and anterior aspects of the shoulder. The patient should be leaning back comfortably against the chair (a chair with arms is ideal) so that they are well supported. Remove anything from the surrounding area in case they faint and fall off the chair; this is rare but we do need to be vigilant.

1 Palpate the following muscles for tightness or soreness: infraspinatus, levator scapulae,

pectoralis major and minor, rhomboid major and minor, supraspinatus, teres major and minor and the trapezius (not illustrated).

2 Needle the main ashi points in the above muscle groups with MA .

3 Insert needles at LI-16 and LI-14 and attach EA clips.

4 Insert needles at jianqian (M-UE-48) and SI-9 and attach EA clips.

5 Needle LI-15 with MA.

6 Add musculoskeletal points with MA: LI-4, Lu-7, St-38.

7 Turn on the EA machine, set the frequency to 90/30Hz DD and carefully turn up the intensity to a point where the patient feels a comfortable tingling or pulsing sensation. Treat with EA for 10 to 20 minutes.

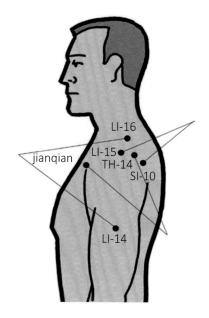

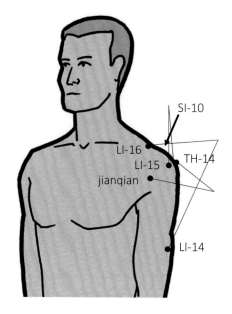

Advanced shoulder treatment

From an EA point of view it is not necessary to differentiate between frozen shoulder and osteo or rheumatoid arthritis of the shoulder as the local treatment is the same for all three.

The advanced treatment is used when the basic treatment has failed or does not seem strong enough.

1 Palpate the following muscles for tightness or soreness: infraspinatus, levator scapulae, pectoralis major and minor, rhomboid major and minor, supraspinatus, teres major and minor and the trapezius. Any tightness in these muscles can restrict mobility of the shoulder.

2 Treat the main ashi points in the above muscle groups with MA .

3 Insert needles at LI-16 and LI-14 and attach one pair of EA clips.

4 Insert needles at jianqian (M-UE-48) and TH-14 and attach another pair of EA clips.

5 Insert needles at LI-15 and SI-10 and attach a third pair of EA clips.

6 Add musculoskeletal points with MA: LI-4, Lu-7, St-38.

7 Add constitutional points with MA.

8 Turn on the EA machine, set the frequency to 90/30Hz DD and carefully turn up the intensity to a point where the patient feels a comfortable tingling or pulsing sensation. Treat with EA for 10 to 20 minutes.

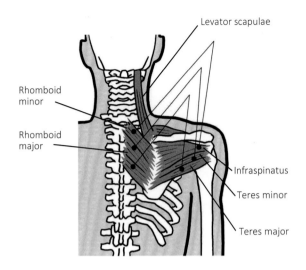
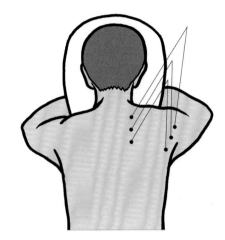

Rhomboids, supraspinatus, infraspinatus and teres

In this presentation the patient is suffering from pain in the right upper back across the shoulder blade; this may, and often does, give rise to neck pain. The muscles involved could be any of the following: rhomboids, supraspinatus, infraspinatus, teres major or minor. When palpating this area we often find tender huatuojiaji points. Other ashi points may also be found along the medial border of the scapula and on the lateral side of the scapula. Rather than using all the ashi points, it is possible to treat all the muscles across the shoulder at the same time by traversing the whole area with three pairs of EA leads. The benefit of this method is that you are placing needles in safe areas of the upper back i.e. not where the rib cage is exposed between the spine and scapula. Moreover fewer needles are used.

1   With the patient in a prone position and their head preferably on a head support, palpate the upper back for tender huatuojiaji points level with the scapula and also palpate along the lateral side of the scapula. Three sets of two points are sufficient to perform this treatment successfully.

2   Place 6 needles in the points selected and attach 3 pairs of EA clips traversing the upper back horizontally.

3   Add musculoskeletal channel points with MA: SI-4, SI-6, BI-63.

4   Add constitutional points with MA.

5   Turn on the EA machine, set the frequency to 6/2Hz DD and carefully turn up the intensity to a point where the patient feels a comfortable tingling or pulsing sensation. Treat with EA for 10 to 20 minutes.

CAUTION

As with all points used in the upper back, the precautions outlined on page 23 should be adopted.

UNDERLYING STRUCTURES

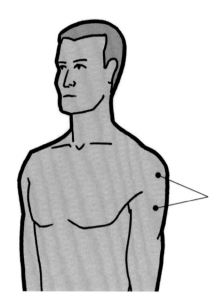

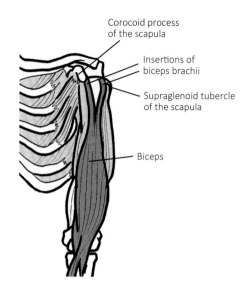

Corocoid process
of the scapula

Insertions of
biceps brachii

Supraglenoid tubercle
of the scapula

Biceps

Biceps brachii

There is often tenderness lateral and superior to jianquan (M-UE-48) at the superior insertions of the biceps brachii and distally along the biceps. If so, apply the following procedure. This treatment can be combined with the other shoulder treatments at the same time.

1 Insert needles at the tender superior insertion of the biceps and a tender point inferior on the biceps muscle. Attach EA clips.

2 Turn on the EA machine, set the frequency to 6/2Hz DD and carefully turn up the intensity to a point where the patient feels a comfortable tingling or pulsing sensation. Treat with EA for 10 to 20 minutes.

CASE STUDY

This 78 year old man presented with severe pain in both shoulders that he had had for some years. He found it difficult to lift his arms above his shoulders. He had a history of rheumatoid arthritis and both knees had been replaced 7 years previously.

EXAMINATION

There seemed to be no obvious problem in the muscles of the shoulders and neck in terms of tightness or soreness. From an EA point of view it is not necessary to differentiate between frozen shoulder and osteo or rheumatoid arthritis of the shoulder as the local treatment is the same for all three.

TREATMENT

1. Applied EA from LI-16(L&R) to LI-14(L&R).

2. Applied EA from jianqian(L&R) to TH-14(L&R).

3. Applied EA from LI-15(L&R) to SI-10(L&R).

4. Added musculoskeletal points with MA: LI-4, Lu-7, St-38.

5. Added constitutional points with MA: Ki-3, St-36, Sp-5.

OUTCOME

The first treatment gave immediate relief and very few follow up treatments were required to maintain improvement. I saw this patient some months later with regards to some other problem and there had been no return of the shoulder problem.

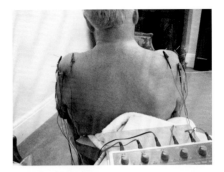

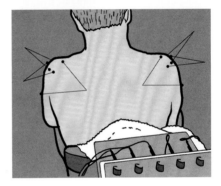

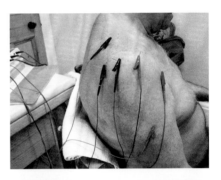

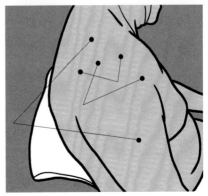

CASE STUDY

This 71 year old man presented with a severe frozen shoulder on the left side that had troubled him for 3 months. The shoulder was extremely painful with very restricted movement.

EXAMINATION

Palpation did not reveal any excessive tightness in the muscles on the front or back of the shoulder so the problem seemed to be mainly in the rotator cuff itself.

TREATMENT

1. Applied EA from LI-16(L) to LI-14(L).

2. Applied EA from jianqian(L) to TH-14(L).

3. Applied EA from LI-15(L) to SI-10(L).

4. Added musculoskeletal points with MA: LI-4, Lu-7, St-38.

5. Added constitutional points with MA: Sp-3, St-36.

OUTCOME

Pain relief was immediate and continued after the first treatment, but further sessions did not improve mobility so treatment was discontinued.

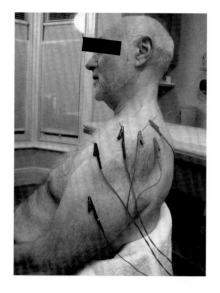

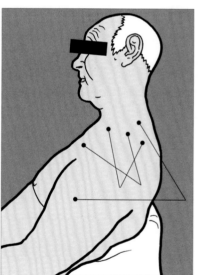

Tennis elbow
& golfer's elbow

8

Tennis elbow or lateral epicondylitis is a painful condition caused by inflammation of the insertion of the extensor muscles of the forearm into the lateral epicondyle. It is thought that the pain is caused by microscopic tears to the tendon between the extensor tendon and the periosteum. Although the term 'epicondylitis' is given to this condition, most histologic findings suggest that there is no acute or chronic inflammation, meaning the pain is probably due to degeneration. It is therefore referred to as tendinopathy rather then tendonitis or angiofibroblastic tendinosis ('Tennis elbow', 2017)[1]. The tendons become painful and damaged through overuse particularly when there is a combination of strenuous movement and gripping tightly with the hand. This is commonly seen with tennis players and labourers wielding a hammer or saw over long periods of time.

The pain is predominantly over the lateral epicondyle although it can radiate along the extensor muscles of the forearm, which are often tender when palpated. The extensor carpi radialis brevis has a key role in the development of the condition although other extensor muscles are often involved. The chronic nature and slow healing of this condition is probably the result of poor blood supply to the tendon and continued use. It may also be exacerbated by the extensor muscles of the forearm being in a chronic state of contraction resulting in stress to the tendon insertions.

Golfer's elbow is a similar condition but affects the medial epicondyle at the insertion of the flexor muscles of the arm. This condition is not exclusive to golfers, but also affects climbers and baseball players. It is the result of excessive gripping by the fingers combined with torsion on the wrist causing stress to the muscles attaching to the medial epicondyle.

Both these conditions can of course arise in people who do not participate in any of these activities.

1. 'Tennis elbow' (2017) *Wikepedia*. Available at https://en.wikipedia.org/wiki/Tennis_elbow (Accessed: 15 November 2017)

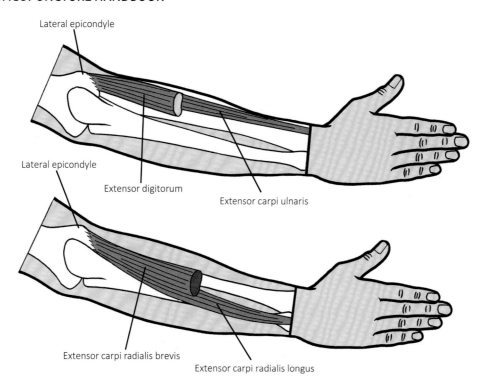

Lateral epicondyle

Lateral epicondyle

Extensor digitorum

Extensor carpi ulnaris

Extensor carpi radialis brevis

Extensor carpi radialis longus

UNDERLYING STRUCTURES TENNIS ELBOW

It is important to understand the underlying structures when treating tennis or golfer's elbow. The first thing to note is that the extensor muscles of the arm insert in the lateral epicondyle and the flexor muscles insert into the medial epicondyle. So it is common to find that the extensor muscles are tight or sore with tennis elbow and the flexor muscles tight or sore with golfer's elbow. Although this is generally the case one must always be aware that muscles that work in opposition to one another may also be causing a problem for one another e.g. tight extensors can cause problems in the flexor muscles leading to golfer's elbow. I therefore recommend a thorough examination of all the muscles of the forearm in both conditions. Occasionally you may find patients who have tight or painful neck or shoulder muscles affecting the nerves coming from the spine which can then cause contraction in the muscles of the forearm. In this situation the muscles of the neck and shoulder also need treating. With many chronic musculoskeletal problems we find a trail of muscle tightness stretching back to the spine.

The underlying structures that are implicated in tennis elbow are the extensor muscles of the forearm which include the extensor carpi radialis brevis, extensor carpi radialis longus, extensor carpi ulnaris and extensor digitorum. In practice it is the extensor carpi radialis brevis that is most commonly the problem. Although it is not of course necessary to identify the muscles by name, it is important to locate the muscles that need treating.

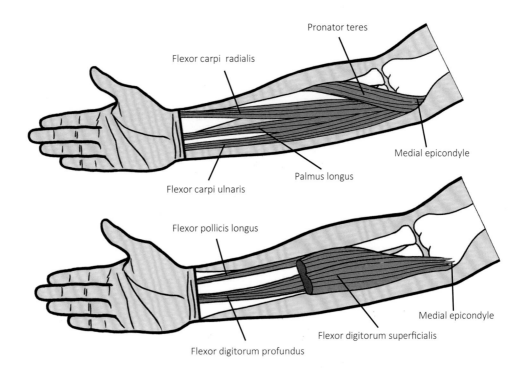

Pronator teres

Flexor carpi radialis

Medial epicondyle

Palmus longus

Flexor carpi ulnaris

Flexor pollicis longus

Medial epicondyle

Flexor digitorum superficialis

Flexor digitorum profundus

UNDERLYING STRUCTURES GOLFER'S ELBOW

The underlying structures that are implicated in golfer's elbow are the flexor muscles of the forearm including flexor carpi radialis, flexor carpi ulnaris, flexor digitorum profundus and flexor digitorum superficialis. If there is tightness in these muscles it is important to check the opposing extensor muscles for tightness and treat them as well.

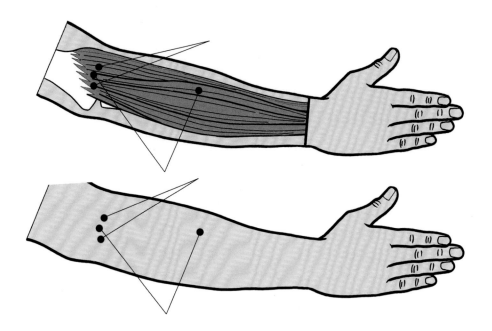

Tennis elbow treatment

1 Palpate the extensor muscles from the lateral epicondyle of the elbow down the forearm to the wrist and take note of any ashi points. Also check the opposing flexor muscles for ashi points.

2 Treat the main ashi points in the above muscle groups with MA.

3 Insert a needle at the most painful point in the tendon at the elbow. Insert another needle in a tender point in the belly of the extensor muscle that seems to be primarily implicated and attach EA clips.

4 Insert a needle either side of the painful point at the insertion of the muscle and attach EA clips.

5 Add musculoskeletal points with MA: TH-5, GB-34, LI-4.

6 Add constitutional points with MA.

7 Turn on the EA machine, set the frequencies to 6/2Hz DD along the muscle and 20/6Hz DD across the tendon - if you only have one machine use 6/2Hz for both - and carefully turn up the intensity to a point where the patient feels a comfortable tingling or pulsing sensation. Treat with EA for 10 to 20 minutes.

NOTE

The above example gives a simple basic treatment; however it may be necessary to address other extensor muscles at the same time in the same way. From a Chinese channel perspective the muscles involved coincide approximately with the SI, TH and LI channels which is useful to know when selecting distal points.

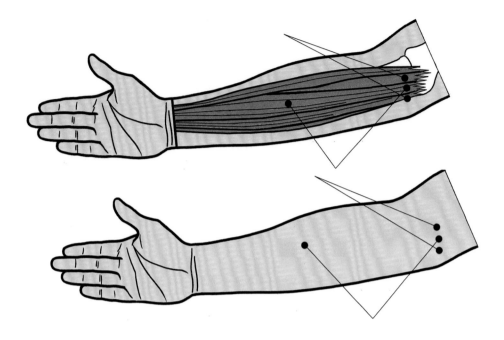

Golfer's elbow treatment

1 Palpate the flexor muscles from the medial epi-condyle of the elbow down the forearm to the wrist and take note of any ashi points. Also check the opposing extensor muscles for ashi points.

2 Treat the main ashi points in the above muscle groups with MA.

3 Insert a needle at the most painful point in the tendon at the elbow. Insert another needle in a tender point in the belly of the flexor muscle that seems to be primarily implicated and attach EA clips.

4 Insert a needle either side of the painful point at the insertion of the muscle and attach a pair of EA clips.

5 Add musculoskeletal points with MA.

6 Add constitutional points with MA.

7 Turn on the EA machine, set the frequencies to 6/2Hz DD along the muscle and 20/6Hz DD across the tendon - if you only have one machine use 6/2Hz for both - and carefully turn up the intensity to a point where the patient feels a comfortable tingling or pulsing sensation. Treat with EA for 10 to 20 minutes.

NOTE

The above example gives a simple basic treatment; however it may be necessary to address other flexor muscles at the same time in the same way.

CASE STUDY

This 55 year old midwife presented with tennis elbow in the left elbow which had been troubling her for several months. She also had osteoarthritis in the second joint of the second finger of her left hand and lower backache that she had had for many years. In this example I will concentrate on the elbow and finger. From a Chinese perspective she was Heart and Kidney yin deficient.

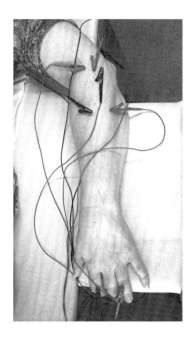

EXAMINATION

The finger joint was not particularly swollen or red. The insertions of the extensor muscles were tender at the lateral epicondyle around LI-11 and also more laterally around the outside of the elbow. The most affected muscles were the extensor carpi radialis brevis and the extensor carpi ulnaris. Identifying the muscles by name is not important: what is important is to identify the tender muscle insertion and the muscle connected to it. There were also tender points along the extensor muscles.

TREATMENT

1. Applied EA along the two affected extensor muscles from their insertion to a tender point along the body of the muscle.

2. Applied EA across the insertion of the extensor muscles at LI-11.

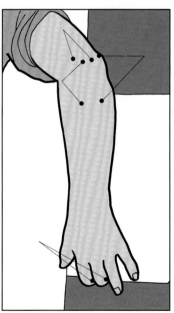

3. Applied EA across the second joint of the second finger.

4. Added musculoskeletal points with MA: LI-4, TH-5.

5. Added constitutional points with MA: Bl-23, GV-14, GV-4, Ht-6, Ki-6.

OUTCOME

After 6 treatments the elbow problem was resolved and the osteoarthritis in the finger was considerably better after only 3 treatments. At her initial consul-

tation she omitted to mention her backache which she thought was untreatable, because she had had it for 20 years; however, after 6 treatments with EA this was also 90% better.

Carpal tunnel syndrome

9

Carpal tunnel syndrome, also called median nerve entrapment neuropathy, is a painful condition where compression of the median nerve that travels through the carpal tunnel causes pain and paraesthesia in the hand. The median nerve innervates the skin of the palmar side of the index finger, the thumb, middle finger and half the ring finger. Compression of this nerve which runs below the flexor retinaculum can cause sensory loss in the fingers and thumb and also atrophy of the thenar muscles. The superficial sensory branch of the median nerve, which provides sensation to the base of the palm, branches proximal to the flexor retinaculum and travels superficial to it so there is no loss of sensation in the palm.

The main symptoms of carpal tunnel syndrome are pain, numbness, and tingling in the thumb, index finger, middle finger, and the radial side of the ring finger. Pain may also extend up the arm. Over time the grip may become weaker and wastage of the thenar muscle at the base of the thumb may occur. The condition is often more painful at night and the patient may report how dangling their arm out of bed or putting their hand behind their head gives some relief. Some patients are encouraged to wear a splint to prevent the hand moving into a flexed position while they are asleep as that exacerbates the problem. The usual treatment for this condition is surgery to open up the carpal tunnel and take pressure off the median nerve. Acupuncture, and especially EA, is effective for treating this condition.

Swelling in the wrist can be caused by overall inflammatory conditions in the body, or more localised inflammation from RSI. Overuse of the flexor muscles can cause a thickening of the tendons running through the carpal tunnel. Another possible cause is localised structural changes to the bones inside the carpal tunnel itself causing the tunnel to narrow. Some sources suggest that median nerve symptoms can arise from compression at the level of the thoracic outlet or in the area where the median nerve passes between the two heads of the pronator teres in the forearm.

From a TCM perspective carpal tunnel syndrome can be caused by dampness, stagnation of Blood or problems with tendons not being nourished.

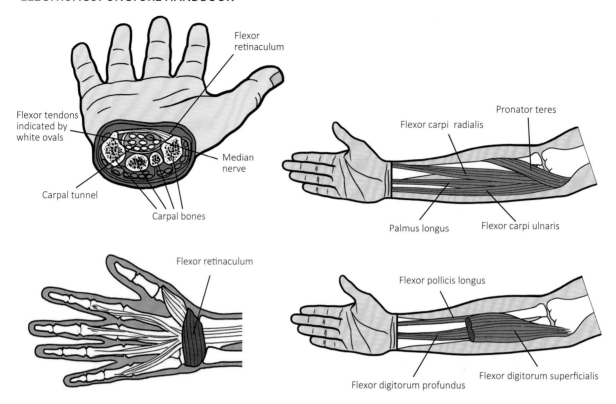

Flexor retinaculum

Flexor tendons indicated by white ovals

Carpal tunnel

Median nerve

Carpal bones

Pronator teres

Flexor carpi radialis

Palmus longus

Flexor carpi ulnaris

Flexor retinaculum

Flexor pollicis longus

Flexor digitorum profundus

Flexor digitorum superficialis

UNDERLYING STRUCTURES

The carpal tunnel is a space in the wrist surrounded on three sides by the carpal bones. The medial side of the carpal tunnel is covered by the flexor retinaculum ligament. The carpal tunnel itself has 9 flexor tendons and the median nerve running through it. If there is any swelling of the tendons then this will ultimately put pressure on the median nerve causing pain and numbness in the fingers.

When treating carpal tunnel syndrome it is important to recognise that some of the problem at the wrist may be caused by tightness in the flexor muscles of the forearm. These include the flexor carpi ulnaris, flexor carpi radialis, flexor digitorum superficialis and profundus, flexor pollicis longus and palmar longus.

It is important to check whether the problem is accompanied by any tightening in the neck muscles as this can affect the nerves supplying the arm muscles.

Although this problem can be related to wider constitutional imbalances, it is often necessary to apply strong local treatment at the wrist to resolve this issue.

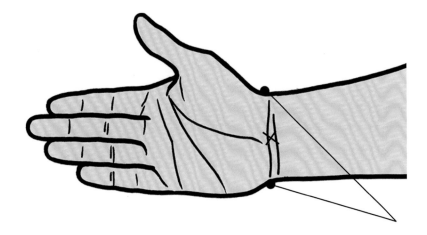

Basic carpal tunnel treatment

1 Commence by checking the neck for tightness in the muscles in case they are impinging on any nerves that could affect the function of the muscles of the forearm. This can be done by following the initial protocol for treating a frozen shoulder (page 41).

2 Needle any ashi points in the neck with MA.

3 With the patient lying on their back palpate and needle any ashi points in the flexor muscles of the forearm with MA.

4 Insert needles in SI-5 and LI-5 using 15mm needles. Attach EA clips.

5 Add musculoskeletal channel points with MA: P-7, GB-34.

6 Add constitutional points with MA.

7 Turn on the EA machine, set the frequency to 20/6Hz DD and carefully turn up the intensity to a point where the patient feels a comfortable tingling or pulsing sensation. Treat with EA for 10 to 20 minutes.

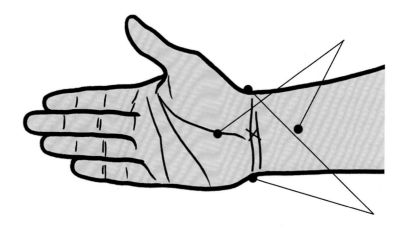

Advanced carpal tunnel treatment

The advanced treatment is used for more severe chronic cases.

1 Follow the protocol for the basic treatment.

2 Insert needles at 1.5cun proximal to P-7 and a point 2cun distal to P-7. This point is in the hollow at the proximal/medial border of the thenar eminence. Attach the clips.

3 Turn on the EA machine, set the frequency to 20/6Hz DD and carefully turn up the intensity to a point where the patient feels a comfortable tingling or pulsing sensation. Treat with EA for 10 to 20 minutes.

NOTE

The purpose of the basic treatment is to pass electricity from one side of the wrist to the other horizontally through the carpal tunnel. In this technique, electricity is also passed through the carpal tunnel in the direction of the flexors. Using both techniques together has a stronger effect in freeing up any stagnation in the carpal tunnel by applying electricity in both directions at the same time.

CASE STUDY

Originally this 80 year old woman came to see me some years ago for severe lower back pain. This time she was barely able to use her right hand because of the increasing stiffness and bony changes that had developed in the finger joints. She was experiencing numbness, pain and tingling in this hand. Whether this condition was arthritis or carpal tunnel syndrome or both is difficult to say.

EXAMINATION

The hand and fingers of the right hand were clearly swollen in comparison to the other. The hand was redder than the other, particularly the fingertips.

TREATMENT

1. Applied EA from SI-5(R) to LI-5(R).

2. Applied EA from a point 1.5cun proximal to P-7(R) to a point approximately 2cun distal to P-7(R).

3. Added P-7(R) with MA.

4. Added constitutional points with MA: Bl-18, Bl-20, Bl-21, Du-8, Du-6, Liv-3, Sp-6, St-36, LI-4, Ren-12.

OUTCOME

Although the acupuncture improved the condition considerably, it did not lead to her regaining the full use of the hand and so she referred herself to the doctor with a view to an operation which I felt would give her more benefit. This case illustrates how important it is to catch this condition in the early stages.

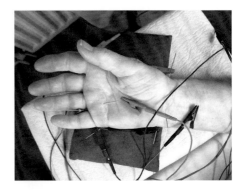

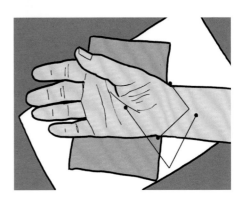

CASE STUDY

This 68 year old self-employed cleaner came to see me complaining of carpal tunnel syndrome, migraines and a stiff neck. She also had menopausal symptoms with severe night sweats. Pulse and tongue diagnosis confirmed that she was suffering from Kidney yin deficiency and Liver yang rising. It was not surprising to see that a combination of the physically repetitive nature of her job and constitutional imbalances had led to a carpal tunnel problem.

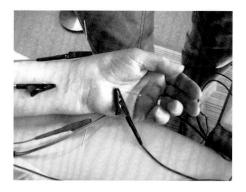

EXAMINATION

On palpating her forearms I noticed a number of ashi points in the flexor muscles. The wrists themselves had gone through bony changes with a peculiar thickening and smoothing of the ulna and radius which I tend to associate with Kidney deficiency. I imagine that the bony changes on the exterior of the wrists had also occurred on their interior, possibly reducing the carpal tunnel size.

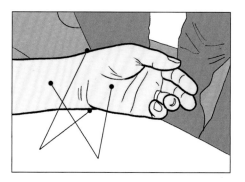

TREATMENT

1. Applied EA from SI-5 to LI-5 on both wrists.

2. Applied EA from a point 1.5cun proximal to P-7 to a point approximately 2cun distal to P-7 on both wrists.

3. Added P-7 with MA on both wrists.

4. Added constitutional points with MA: Bl-18, Bl-23, Du-14, Ki-6, TH-5, GB-20, GB-43, Liv-2, Ren-7, Ren-4.

OUTCOME

By the 4th treatment the headaches and night sweats had stopped. By the 9th treatment the carpal tunnel symptoms were 70% better and, by the 11th, 100% better. This was 5 years ago. Since then she has been coming once every 6 to 8 weeks which keeps her symptoms in check and she has been able to continue working.

Fingers & thumbs
osteoarthritis & rheumatoid arthritis

10

Osteoarthritis and rheumatoid arthritis of the thumb and fingers usually start with feelings of stiffness in the joints which can be associated with particular weather conditions i.e. cold or damp. The condition can be caused or exacerbated by certain activities where the hands are constantly exposed to cold water. As it develops, the joints become painful and swollen, sometimes with bony changes. Over a period of time the fingers can become very deformed and misaligned. The fingers and thumbs lie at the extremities of the body with very little muscle or fat protecting them and so are particularly vulnerable to external factors.

Another factor that may possibly exacerbate arthritis of the fingers is carpal tunnel syndrome. Any compression or constriction in the carpal tunnel can impede the circulation to the fingers and thumb leading to colder poorly nourished fingers. This will reduce the body's ability to repair any damage to the finger joints.

From a TCM perspective most arthritis is the result of an underlying constitutional weakness that allows external pathogens, usually climatic in nature, to invade the body. Sometimes the treatment of that underlying metabolic imbalance is not enough to improve or resolve arthritis in the hands without using localised EA treatment of individual finger or thumb joints and possibly the wrist.

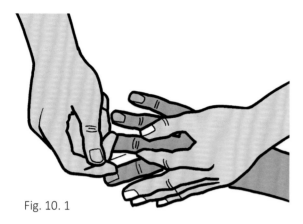
Fig. 10. 1

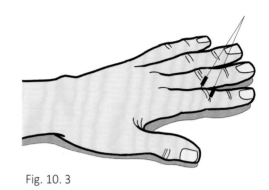
Fig. 10. 3

Finger joint treatment

1 When treating the finger joints there are two methods of insertion you can employ. The first is performed without a needle tube. With this method it is important that the hand is placed firmly palm down, fingers splayed out (Fig. 10. 1). This can be done with the patient lying face up, with palms face down on the couch. Press down firmly with your left hand on the back of the patient's hand and grip their finger proximal to the joint being treated. Grip it tightly to make it feel uncomfortable; this will reduce the pain felt by the needle being inserted. Always use short 15mm needles. The second method for a relatively painless insertion is to use a needle tube and press the side of the end of the tube against the side of the finger joint so it creates a little discomfort; this likewise will distract the patient from the insertion of the needle.

2 Place a needle on either side of the joint to be treated and attach EA clips. It is important that the needles are oppo-

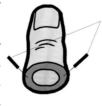
Fig. 10. 2

site each other either side of the finger and just under the skin without penetrating the joint. With practice this can be done swiftly and fairly painlessly (Figs. 10.2, 10.3). This positioning maximises the possibility of the electricity passing through the joint itself.

Very often a patient may have a number of joints affected on one hand. In this situation you can treat up to three joints at a time (Fig. 10. 4). Anything over this becomes impractical with too many wires and clips. It is also rather uncomfortable for the patient when so many fingers are treated simultaneously. When treating two joints next to one another it is important that one pair of leads and needles don't

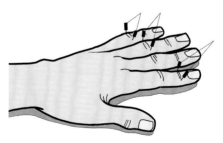
Fig. 10. 4

touch the adjacent ones as this will affect the direction of the electrical current; so I suggest that cotton wool is placed between the needles or clips to prevent any needle or clip touching another needle or clip (Fig. 10. 5).

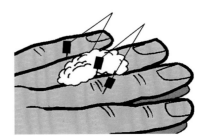

Fig. 10. 5

3 Apply musculoskeletal points with MA: baxie, TH-5, LI-4.

4 Add constitutional points with MA.

5 Turn on the EA machine, set the frequency to 90/30Hz DD and carefully turn up the intensity to a point where the patient feels a comfortable tingling or pulsing sensation. Treat with EA for 10 to 20 minutes.

Thumb joint treatment

The carpometacarpal joint can be treated in much the same way as the fingers, but the metacarpophalangeal joint (Fig. 10. 6) should be approached with a slightly different needle technique. As with most of the treatments in this book it is of paramount importance that the needles are placed diametrically opposite each other when treating joints. With the metacarpophalangeal joint it is relatively easy to direct the needles towards the joint because there is more tissue surrounding it than the finger joints. Before placing the needles, hold the joint with your thumb and forefinger to be sure that you are placing the needles diametrically opposite each other on either side of the joint.

As with all techniques in this book it is important to address the underlying constitutional problem from a TCM perspective with MA.

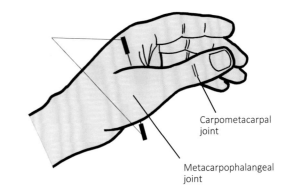

Carpometacarpal joint

Metacarpophalangeal joint

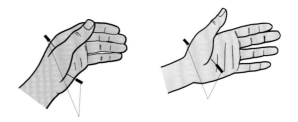

Fig. 10. 6

CASE STUDY

This 54 year old female I have treated intermittently over the last 20 years for a variety of problems including migraine, neck pain, constipation and post hysterectomy exhaustion. This time she presented with arthritis of the fingers with pain, stiffness and bony changes to the distal joints of the first and second fingers of her right hand and the second finger of her left hand; also numbness and tingling in her right hand. My suspicion is that arthritis of the fingers can be exacerbated by carpal tunnel syndrome: if the patient is experiencing numbness and tingling in the hand I treat both conditions simultaneously.

EXAMINATION

On palpation of the flexors of the forearms there were no tender or sore points. On examination of the neck there was tightness in the levator scapulae on the right side.

TREATMENT

As you can see from the picture the patient is lying face down on the couch with the hands supported on a stool. The reason for this is that I am treating the neck and back at the same time as the fingers.

1. Applied EA across the joints of the 1st and 2nd fingers of the right hand and the 2nd finger of the left hand.

2. Applied EA from the superior to the inferior borders of the levator scapulae on the right hand side.

3. Applied EA from SI-5(R) to LI-5(R).

4. Added no other musculoskeletal points.

5. Added constitutional points with MA: Bl-18, Bl-23, TH-5, GB-39, Liv-3.

OUTCOME

The numbness and tingling in the right hand and pain and stiffness in the fingers of both hands were 80% better after the first treatment and had gone after the third treatment. The patient is still coming for treatment on a monthly basis to prevent a recurrence of the problem.

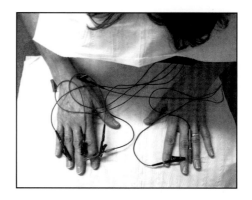

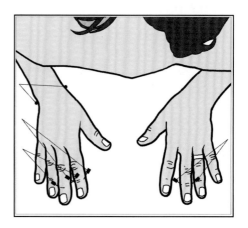

CASE STUDY

This 69 year old man first came to see me in 1996 with extreme stress due to his job as the deputy head of a school. He was suffering from severe vertigo and tinnitus. Because he initially benefited from treatment he decided to see me every 2 or 3 months. He had remarkably well-balanced pulses in all positions apart from the Lung position. Since 1996 treating the Lung had been the main focus of my treatments and he generally remained very well. In 2009 he complained about pain and stiffness in the metacarpophalangeal joint in both thumbs. The location was not of course a surprise in view of his weak Lung qi, but it was surprising that the treatment had not averted this problem. MA didn't resolve the problem so I used EA.

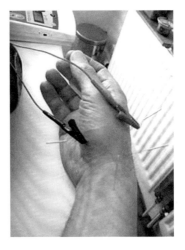

TREATMENT

1. Applied EA across the metacarpophalangeal joint of both thumbs.

2. Added musculoskeletal point with MA: LI-5.

3. Added constitutional points with MA: Bl-13, Ren-17, Lu-7, LI-4, St-36.

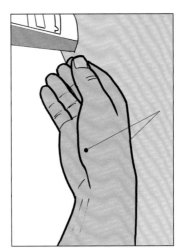

OUTCOME

The thumbs showed immediate improvement on the first EA treatment. Over the years I have occasionally had to apply EA to the thumbs, and they remain pain free.

Lower back pain
sciatica, disc narrowing & disc herniation

11

Chronic lower back pain is probably one of the prices we pay for being bipeds. Problems are not surprising when our spine, which could be described as 27 bones piled on top of one another interleaved with soft cartilaginous discs, connects our heavy upper body to a two legged base. The vertebral column is under tremendous stress throughout the day; so much so that the spine can shrink by 2cm over a twelve hour period as the discs become slowly compressed by the weight of the body. It is natural and inevitable for some disc narrowing to occur during the day, but if this narrowing becomes excessive we begin to experience nerve entrapment and pain; this can manifest as pain in our backs and pain running down our arms and/or legs.

Narrowing of the vertebral discs can also occur as a result of chronic contraction of the vertebral muscles, injury to the back or degeneration from ageing. Being overweight and hard physical work can both exacerbate back pain.

Poor posture can lead to excessive tension and muscle contraction, particularly in the lumbar area. In addition, sitting in a sedentary position for long periods can cause the muscles to be in an unrelenting state of tension that can then affect the lumbar discs. Sitting can also cause contraction and shortening of the psoas muscles, which are then overly tight when the body is in a standing position. Unsurprisingly disc problems usually occur in the lower back which is the part under most stress being positioned at the base of the spine.

From a TCM perspective underlying Kidney deficiency can directly cause back pain. Spleen deficiency can lead to the accumulation of fluid in the lower back causing stiffness or general muscular weakness with the inability to lift the head. Liver stagnation can lead to the back muscles being overly tight. Lung deficiency may cause kyphosis that could lead to extra strain on the lumbar region. Other reasons for back pain include external invasion of cold, damp or heat. However the vast majority of back pain, in my experience, is muscular in origin and is best treated in a musculoskeletal way.

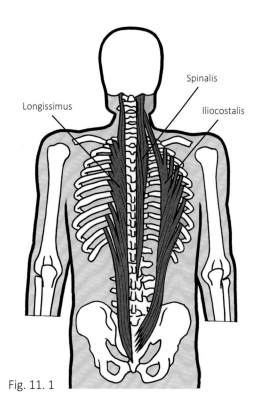

Fig. 11. 1

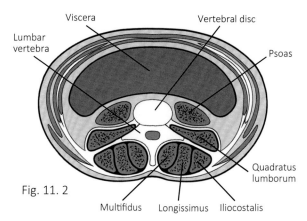

Fig. 11. 2

CROSS SECTION OF THE LUMBAR TORSO

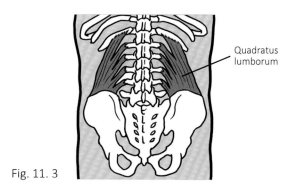

Fig. 11. 3

UNDERLYING STRUCTURES

The important underlying structures of the back are of course the spine itself and the muscles of the back. At the superficial layer are the erector spinae muscles: these include the iliocostalis, longissimus and spinalis (Fig. 11. 1). The iliocotalis and longissimus run from the neck to the sacrum and the spinalis muscles run from the neck to the beginning of the lumbar spine. Underlying these muscles in the lumbar region laterally are the quadratus lumborum (Figs. 11. 2 and 11.3) which attach to the 12th rib, the transverse processes of the lumbar spine from L1 to L4 and the iliac crest. Beneath the erector spinae muscles along the spine are the multifidus and rotatores muscles: these are groups of short muscles connecting one vertebra to the next. The deepest muscles in the back

are the psoas which lie lateral to the lumbar spine. The superior attachments are to the transverse processes of the lumbar vertebrae from L1 to L5 and to the vertebral bodies of T12 to L5; the inferior attachments are to the lesser trochanter of the femur.

INITIAL EXAMINATION

When treating back problems it is easy to assume that the spine is at the posterior of the body because we can easily palpate the spinous processes of the spine from the back; however, it is more helpful to think of the spinal column as situated centrally in the body. Fig. 11. 2 is a cross section of the lumbar torso and clearly shows the spinal column positioned centrally, surrounded by the spinal muscles. It also

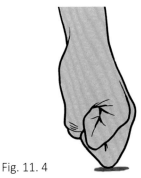

Fig. 11. 4

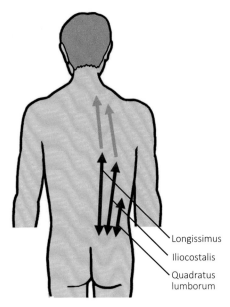

Fig. 11. 5

illustrates the depths we need to reach in order to affect the deep muscles in the back.

When palpating the lumbar muscles it is often necessary to palpate with considerable pressure in order to find the ashi points. This can be quite a strain on the thumb or finger joints; I therefore use the protruding second joint of the second finger while holding the hand in a fist (Fig. 11. 4). In this position you can apply very focused controlled pressure on specific areas. Also, with the finger joint pressed into the back, the other bent finger joints rest naturally on the back, preventing the hand from slipping off any tight bands of muscle which can be uncomfortable for the patient. At first it seems a bit ham-fisted but actually you can develop considerable accuracy and sensitivity in the bent finger.

With the patient face down, palpate down the back from the neck to the lumbar region, taking note of any ashi points or chronic tightness in any of the back muscles such as the iliocostalis, longissimus and spinalis. When palpating the lumbar region, first examine the quadratus lumborum. Also palpate the huatuojiaji (M-BW-35) points in the lumbar region to reveal any tightness in the superficial and deep muscles. Any tender points in the back muscles can be potentially used for treatment with EA or MA. Ideally we are looking to find a band of tightness that includes ashi points running down the back in order to use EA successfully.

BANDS OF MUSCLES

In view of the fact that the back muscles are not completely distinct entities but enmeshed with each other it is not always possible to have a clear-cut diagnosis of distinct muscle groups. The bands of tightness may well be the result of a number of muscle groups interacting together causing a single band. It is important to palpate the bands accurately in order to be effective. These bands or tight cords in the back fall into three categories (Fig. 11. 5).

1. Bands close to the spinal column along the huatuojiaji points in the lumbar region are the longissimus muscles.
2. Bands running along the inner or outer Bladder channel starting superior to the iliac crest and continuing above the 12th rib are the iliocostalis muscles.
3. Bands running along the outer Bladder line commencing at the superior border of the iliac crest and stopping below the 12th rib are the quadratus lumborum muscles.

POSITIONING THE NEEDLES

When positioning the pairs of EA needles one should aim at running along the fibres of the muscles and not across them. If, for instance, there are tender points at the superior and inferior aspects of the quadratus lumborum, EA should be applied from top to bottom of the muscle. Applying EA above and below the areas of soreness in a particular muscle can also be effective as long as the points lie in the muscle itself. The ashi points in between the EA points can be needled manually.

NEEDLE DEPTH

The recommended depth for needling the huatuojiaji (M-BW-35) points in the lumbar region is between 0.5 and 1cun; in practice, I often needle up to 1.5 cun, and with obese patients up to 3cun. In order to affect the deep intervertebral muscles such as the multifidus and the rotatores, deep insertion is necessary. I have needled to these depths for a number of years without any adverse effects. I avoid any deep needling of the huatuojiaji points above T12. On a patient of average weight I generally use 50mm needles for the huatuojiaji points at L4, L5 and QL5, QL6, QL7 and QL8 (QL refers to quadratus lumborum Fig. 11. 8). For overweight patients I may have to use up to 75mm needles. It is important to make sure that the needles are inserted into the muscle and not just into the fat layer.

For any other points in the lumbar region below the 12th rib in a patient of average weight I tend to use 30mm needles.

It is worth noting that even at these depths the tips of the needles are only lateral to the spinal cord and not lateral to the discs themselves (Figs. 11 .6 and 11. 7). This treatment relies on releasing any tightness in the muscles that the needles can reach posterior to the transverse processes of the spine. It is difficult to ascertain the depth of influence of the

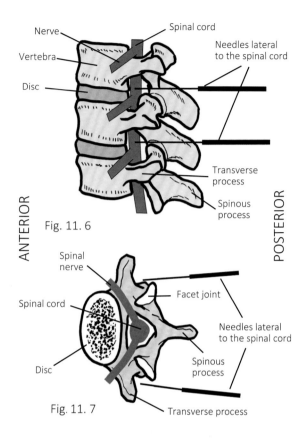

Fig. 11. 6

Fig. 11. 7

electricity beyond the tip of the needle but I suspect that it does not just end at the tip but penetrates deeper into the body.

NEEDLING TECHNIQUE

It is important to approach deep needling with caution and patience, with a slow insertion of the needle, to avoid getting deqi. If you do inadvertently get deqi you might initiate a strong contraction in the muscle and cause unnecessary pain to the patient. Because we are using electrical stimulation it is unnecessary to elicit deqi; in fact we should consciously aim at avoiding it, particularly with tight painful backs. When needling very tight sore muscles we should carefully and slowly insert the needle incrementally without rotating, pushing the needle in a couple of millimetres, then pausing and pushing the needle in another couple more millimetres. We may have to leave the needle a couple of minutes before proceeding if the patient feels discomfort. If we are too quick at this point we may lose the patient's confidence. Sometimes the muscles of the back are so tight to begin with that we may only be able to penetrate the surface in the initial treatments, but as the muscles relax and become softer we can penetrate more deeply. With acute spasm in the back it may be inadvisable to begin treatment with EA.

QUADRATUS LUMBORUM NOMENCLATURE

Fig. 11. 8 illustrates a shorthand way of recording the common ashi points in the quadratus lumborum.

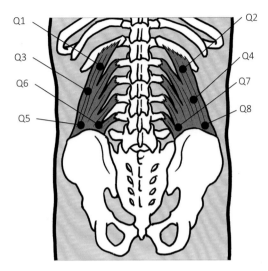

Fig. 11. 8

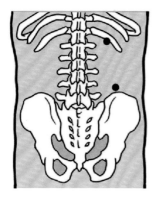 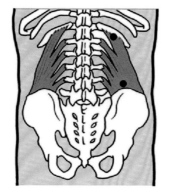 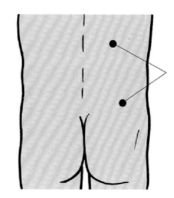

Quadratus lumborum treatment

The diagram above illustrates probably the most common back pain we will encounter which is a problem with the quadratus lumborum. The black dots represent the points of tenderness on palpation and possible sites for treatment. In this example the problem is one-sided but it can be bilateral. This is diagnosed by palpating the area between the lowest rib and the top of the iliac crest. Typically there are eight possible points that may be tender. It is best to choose points on the superior and inferior borders of the quadratus lumborum to apply EA, so that the flow of electricity runs along the muscle fibres, for example QL1 to QL5 or QL2 to QL8 (see Fig. 11. 8). In this way the electricity runs through the whole of the muscle. QL3 and QL4 can be included with MA.

1 Palpate the lumbar region on the side of the pain; establish the tender or sore points on the superior and inferior borders of the quadratus lumborum.

2 Insert needles in the ashi points on the superior insertion of the quadratus lumborum below the 12th rib and the inferior insertion just above the iliac crest. Attach EA clips.

3 Needle any other local ashi points with MA.

4 Add musculoskeletal points with MA: Bl-26(R), Du-4, Du-3, SI-3(R), SI-6(R), Bl-40(R), Bl-60(R), Bl-63(R), GB-34(R).

5 Add constitutional points with MA.

6 Turn on the EA machine, set the frequency to 6/2Hz DD and carefully turn up the intensity to a point where the patient feels a comfortable tingling or pulsing sensation. Treat with EA for 10 to 20 minutes.

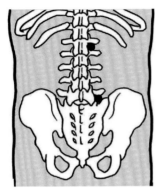 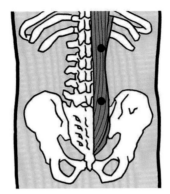 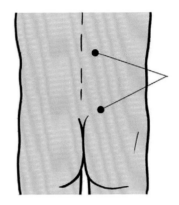

Longissimus treatment

In the scenario above we can see that there are points of tenderness closer to the spine than in the previous example. These points coincide with the huatuojiaji points and relate to the longissimus muscle primarily, although there may be some involvement of the deeper muscles - multifidus and rotatores. In practice we often find that the points lateral to L4 and L5 are the most tender. When treating these points with EA it is better to apply EA above the tender points, say from T12 or L1 to L5, and needle L4 manually. The reason for this is that there is probably some contraction of the muscle above the area of tenderness. By including this portion of the muscle you are freeing up all areas of possible contraction. In some cases it may be necessary to go much further up the back if the tightness of the muscle extends higher up.

1. Palpate the lumbar spine lateral to the spine on the huatuojiaji points and establish where the points of tenderness are.

2. Insert needles above and below this area along the spine. You may find that L4 and L5 are particularly sore; therefore apply EA from a point above this area e.g. L1 to L5. Attach EA clips.

3. Needle any other local ashi points with MA.

4. Add musculoskeletal points with MA:
Bl-26(R), Du-4, Du-3, SI-3(R), SI-6(R), Bl-40(R), Bl-60(R), Bl-63(R), GB-34(R).

5. Treat constitutional points with MA.

6. Turn on the EA machine, set the frequency to 6/2Hz DD and carefully turn up the intensity to a point where the patient feels a comfortable tingling or pulsing sensation. Treat with EA for 10 to 20 minutes.

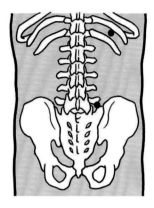 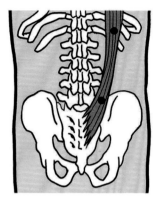 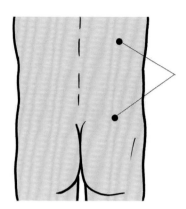

Iliocostalis treatment

Sometimes, upon palpating the lumbar region, we find that the bands of tight, sore muscle continue above the 12th rib; this indicates that it is not primarily the quadratus lumborum that is the cause, but the iliocostalis.

1   Palpate the lumbar and mid back lateral to the spine along the iliocostalis muscles to establish where the points of tenderness are.

2   Insert needles at the superior and inferior aspects of the iliocostalis muscle on the affected side. Attach EA clips.

3   Needle any other local ashi points with MA.

4   Add musculoskeletal points with MA:
Bl-26(R), Du-4, Du-3, SI-3(R), SI-6(R), Bl-40(R), Bl-60(R), Bl-63(R), GB-34(R).

5   Treat constitutional points with MA.

6   Turn on the EA machine, set the frequency to 6/2Hz DD and carefully turn up the intensity

to a point where the patient feels a comfortable tingling or pulsing sensation. Treat with EA for 10 to 20 minutes.

Narrowed or herniated disc treatment

When treating disc problems it is helpful to ascertain which disc or discs are involved; MRI scans can be useful in establishing this because, with some chronic disc problems, large areas of the lower back may be tender and so palpation is not a diagnostic option.

If an MRI is not available then you will have to rely on palpation and the symptoms to reveal where the disc or discs are damaged. Sometimes, as in the example illustrated to the right, there is no tenderness or soreness in any of the lumbar muscles but there is tenderness to the right and left of L5. In this scenario one only needs to apply EA across the disc in question. Treatment can have a freeing effect on the longissimus, multifidus and rotatores and also have a stimulating healing effect on the disc itself.

This particular treatment can be helpful after disc surgery when the patient is still suffering from pain that may well be more related to scar tissue than the original problem.

CROSSING THE SPINE

It is widely believed that crossing the spine with EA may be dangerous, particularly in the upper back, as it could adversely affect the heart and theoretically any other organ by affecting the nerves emerging from the spine. The spinal cord ends around the L1/L2 vertebral level, forming a structure known as the conus medullaris; it is considered safe to cross the spine inferior to L2. Most disc problems occur below L2.

Sometimes more than one disc is herniated or damaged. In this situation you can apply EA across multiple discs. It may be the case that the intervertebral muscles are also tight, which of course may be the cause of the narrowing of the discs in the first place. In this situation you will have to apply EA

across the spine to treat the discs themselves and also stimulate the muscles either side of the spine in two stages.

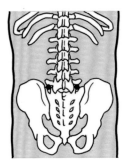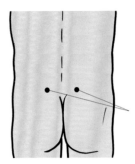

This diagram illustrates how to treat the disc at L5.

1 Establish which disc/discs are involved either by palpation and/or from an MRI scan. If an MRI scan is not available you will have to rely on palpation and the symptomatology.

2 Insert needles in huatuojiaji points inferior to L5. Attach EA clips crossing the spine.

3 Needle any other local ashi points with MA.

4 Add musculoskeletal points with MA: Bl-26, Du-4, Du-3, Bl-40, Bl-60.

5 Treat constitutional points with MA.

6 Turn on the EA machine, set the frequency to 20/6Hz DD and carefully turn up the intensity to a point where the patient feels a comfortable tingling or pulsing sensation. Treat with EA for 10 to 20 minutes.

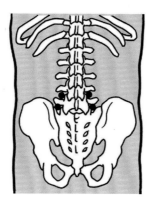 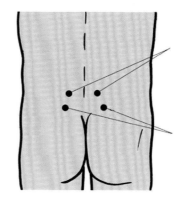

Narrowed or herniated discs inferior to L4 and L5

The above diagram illustrates how to treat more than one disc problem. Commonly it is the discs at L4 and/or L5 that are affected.

1 Establish which discs are involved either by palpation and/or from an MRI scan. If an MRI scan is not available you will have to rely on palpation and the symptomatology.

2 Insert needles in huatuojiaji points inferior to L4 and L5. Attach 2 pairs of EA clips crossing the spine.

3 Needle any other local ashi points with MA.

4 Add musculoskeletal points with MA: Bl-26, Du-4, Du-3, Bl-40, Bl-60.

5 Treat constitutional points with MA.

6 Turn on the EA machine, set the frequency to 20/6Hz DD and carefully turn up the intensity to a point where the patient feels a comfortable tingling or pulsing sensation. Treat with EA for 10 to 20 minutes.

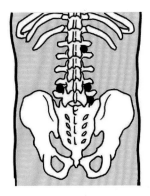 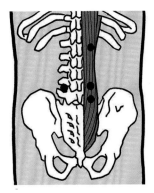 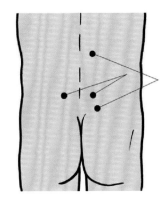

Narrowed or herniated disc inferior to L4 and tightness in the lumbar longissimus muscle on the right

In the above diagram we have a scenario where there is a disc problem at L4 and also tightness in the longissimus muscle on the right hand side of the spine. In this situation we can treat both problems simultaneously.

1 Establish which disc is the problem either by palpation and/or from an MRI scan. If an MRI scan is not available you will have to rely on palpation and the symptomatology.

2 Palpate along the longissimus muscle on the right side of the spine to locate the ashi points superior and inferior to the herniated disc. Insert needles at points superior and inferior to the affected area of the longissimus muscle. Attach EA clips.

3 Insert needles in huatuojiaji points inferior to L4 on the left and right of the spine. Attach EA clips crossing the spine.

4 Needle any local ashi points with MA.

5 Add musculoskeletal points with MA: Bl-26(R), Du-4, Du-3, SI-3(R), SI-6(R), Bl-40(R), Bl-60(R), Bl-63(R), GB-34(R).

6 Add constitutional points with MA.

7 Turn on the EA machine, set the frequencies to 6/2Hz DD along the muscle and 20/6Hz DD across the disc - if you only have one machine use 6/2Hz for both - and carefully turn up the intensity to a point where the patient feels a comfortable tingling or pulsing sensation. Treat with EA for 10 to 20 minutes.

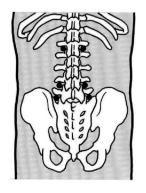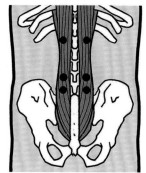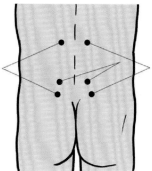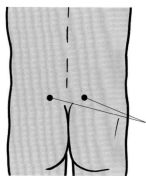

Narrow or herniated discs inferior to L4 and L5 & tightness in the lumbar longissimus muscles bilaterally

In the above diagram we have a scenario where there is a disc problem inferior to L4 and L5 and also tightness in the longissimus muscles on both sides. As we are using the huatuojiaji points inferior to L5 when treating the longissimus muscles we cannot use these points simultaneously to treat the disc below L5. We therefore need to treat the L5 disc after we have treated the longissimus muscles. This means that the treatment is done in two stages. This can of course be achieved by simply moving the clips without having to re-needle.

1 Establish which discs are the problem either by palpation and/or from an MRI scan. If an MRI scan is not available you will have to rely on palpation and the symptomatology. Also palpate the longissimus muscles either side of the spine to establish where the ashi points are before commencing any needling.

2 Insert 4 needles in huatuojiaji points inferior to L4 and L5 bilaterally. Attach EA clips at L4.

3 Insert 2 needles at points superior to the affected areas of the longissimus muscles. Attach EA clips from these points to the huatuojiaji points at L5.

4 Needle any other local ashi points with MA. Add musculoskeletal points with MA: Bl-26, Du-4, Du-3, SI-3, Bl-40, Bl-60, GB-34. Add constitutional points with MA.

5 Apply EA for 10 to 20 minutes horizontally across L4, 20/6Hz DD, and vertically along the longissimus muscles, 6/2Hz DD, being careful to only turn up the intensity to a point where the patient feels a comfortable or pulsing sensation. If you only have one EA machine use 6/2Hz for both. Turn off EA machine.

6 Remove the EA clip from the right superior longissimus and attach to the left of L5 and apply EA for 10 to 20 minutes across L5 20/6 Hz DD, being careful to only turn up the intensity to a point where the patient feels a comfortable or pulsing sensation.

POSTERIOR OF THE BODY

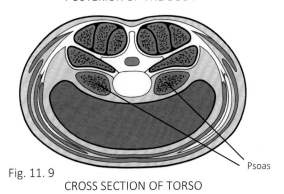

Fig. 11. 9

CROSS SECTION OF TORSO

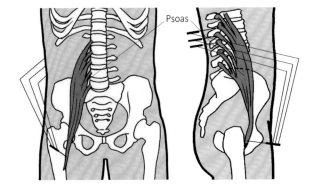

Psoas

Psoas treatment

Although many people claim to be able to treat the psoas muscle with acupuncture, I question the effectiveness of the two approaches I have come across. One technique involves using stomach points on the abdomen, another involves threading needles between the inside of the pelvic girdle and the abdomen into the psoas. The first I thought implausible, the second dangerous and uncomfortable.

The psoas muscles are sandwiched between the anterior of the quadratus lumborum and posterior of the abdominal viscera (Fig. 11. 9). The superior attachments are connected to the transverse processes of the lumbar vertebrae L1 to L5 and also the lumbar vertebrae themselves from T12 to L5; the inferior attachments are connected to the lesser trochanter of the femur.

The psoas muscles are often implicated in back pain particularly when a patient experiences pain and stiffness when trying to stand up from a sitting position. They tend to get stuck in a stooped posture as the psoas muscles can become shortened when people stay seated for a long time. Shortening of the psoas tilts the pelvis forward increasing lordosis in the lumbar spine which can also cause back pain.

1 This treatment is best performed with the patient lying on their side or sitting on a stool facing the couch with their forearms supported on the couch. If both sides need treating then it is more efficient to have them seated. If the psoas is tight on the left side insert needles at the huatuojiaji points at L1, L2 and L3.

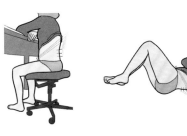

2 Palpate for an ashi point in the area inferior and medial to St-31 on the left leg and insert another needle here. Attach the 3 EA clips from the points on the back to this needle. **It is important to have all the red or black leads together at the front or the back so that the lead colours are not mixed.**

3 Turn on the EA machine, 6/2 Hz DD and carefully turn up the intensity to a point where the patient feels a comfortable tingling or pulsing sensation. Treat with EA for 10 to 20 minutes.

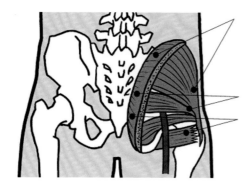 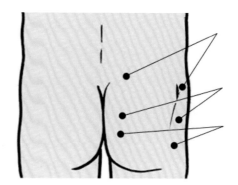

Tightness in the muscles of the buttocks

In this example there is tightness in the muscles of the right buttock. Any of the following muscles could be involved: gluteus maximus and medius, piriformis, gemellus superior and inferior and obturator internus. Osteoarthritis of the hip joint can also cause the muscles to be tight. Tightness can cause hip, buttock and sciatica pain.

1 With the patient in a prone position palpate the lateral edge of the sacrum and the lateral side of the buttock for ashi points. Three sets of two points are sufficient to perform this treatment successfully.

2 Place 6 needles in the points selected and attach the EA clips in 3 pairs traversing the buttock.

3 Add musculoskeletal points with MA: Bl-54, GB-30.

4 Add constitutional points with MA.

5 Turn on the EA machine, set the frequency to 6/2Hz DD and carefully turn up the intensity to a point where the patient feels a comfortable tingling or pulsing sensation. Treat with EA for 10 to 20 minutes.

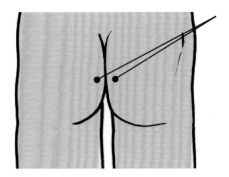 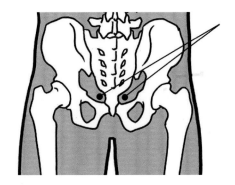

Pain in the coccyx

Pain in the coccyx is called coccydynia and is often the result of an initial injury developing into chronic pain. Sitting down, which is painful, can exacerbate the problem.

1   Place one 75mm needle either side of the coccygeal joint just superior to Bl-35. Attach EA clips.

2   Add musculoskeletal points with MA: Bl-54, Bl-60.

3   Add constitutional points with MA.

4   Turn on the EA machine, set the frequency to 20/6Hz DD and carefully turn up the intensity to a point where the patient feels a comfortable tingling or pulsing sensation. Treat with EA for 10 to 20 minutes.

THE CAT

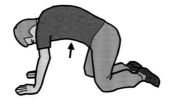

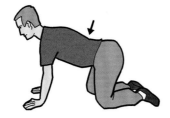

THE TWIST

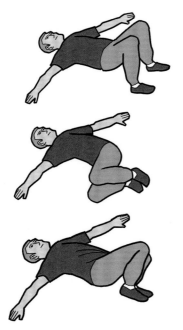

BASIC BACK EXERCISES

The two essential exercises I recommend are both yoga exercises. Both are safe and do not overly load the back muscles as can happen with many back-strengthening exercises. In my experience with chronic back pain the important thing is to first relax the back and free the muscles, tendons and bones. These 2 exercises loosen the back in two planes: the cat frees the posterior and anterior aspects of the spine and the twist frees the muscles laterally by rotation.

CAT

Adopt a position on all fours with your arms and knees a shoulder width apart. Gently tilt the pelvis under, drawing the pubic bone towards the chin while lowering the head. Then tilt your bottom and head towards the ceiling while lowering and curving the lower back down towards the floor. Continue this movement slowly 24 times. It is helpful to synchronise the breath with the movement, breathing in as you tilt the head up and breathing out as you arch the back up. It is important not to strain the back by going to the full stretch in either direction. The emphasis should be on gently mobilising the back rather than stretching excessively.

TWIST

Lie on your back with the arms spread out to the side palms down. Bend the knees and place the feet flat on the floor. The feet and knees can be either shoulder width apart or together so that they are touching at knee and ankle. Slowly lower the knees to one side, keeping the upper back flat on the floor. Then lift the knees back to the central position and lower to the other side. Repeat this exercise 12 times to each side.

Again with this exercise it is important not to over stretch the back but to gently mobilise it. This rotational movement helps stretch the large muscles of the lumbar region and also the smaller intervertebral muscles.

The exercises should be done initially 3 times a day and then a minimum of twice a day, preferably morning and evening.

CASE STUDY

This 58 year old male presented with sciatica running down the back of the right leg. He had been in pain for 6 months.

EXAMINATION

Palpation revealed ashi points at L3, L4 and L5 on the longissimus muscle on the right side but no tightness in the quadratus lumborum.

TREATMENT

1. Applied EA from L1 to L5 on the right side.

2. Added L3 and L4 with MA on the right side.

3. Added musculoskeletal points with MA: QL4, Bl-40(R), GB-34(R) and 3 ashi points on the right iliotibial band.

4. Added constitutional points with MA: Bl-20, Bl-23, Du-6, Du-4, Du-3, Ki-3, Sp-3.

OUTCOME

After the 3rd treatment the sciatica was 70% better; after the 5th treatment the problem seemed to be fully resolved and it was suggested that the patient came back if his symptoms returned.

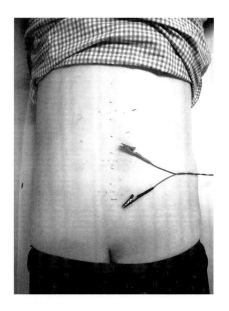

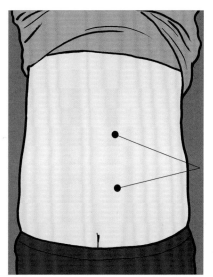

CASE STUDY

This 47 year old male presented with lower back pain that he had had for the previous 12 months. The problem began after a long haul flight when his back went into spasm. Physiotherapy and chiropractic treatment had not significantly reduced his back pain.

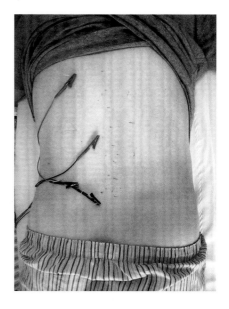

EXAMINATION

On palpation the back was tight in the left lumbar area, particularly the huatuojiaji points from L3 to L5, and also along the iliocostalis on the left side. His Kidney pulses were weak and he tended to get hot at night; the tongue was normal, pink with no coat. From a TCM perspective he was suffering from Kidney yin deficiency.

TREATMENT

1. Applied EA from L1 to L5 on the left side.

2. Applied EA on the iliocostalis muscle, level with T10, to a point superior to the iliac crest on the left side.

3. Added musculoskeletal points with MA: Bl-40(L), GB-34(L).

4. Added constitutional points with MA: Bl-23, Ki-3 and Ki-6.

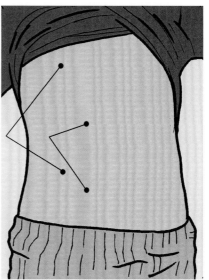

OUTCOME

After two treatments his back moved more freely and he was in less pain. After 5 treatments the condition was much improved with some residual stiffness in the morning. The treatment was supplemented by the two exercises recommended in this book.

CASE STUDY

This 80 year old lady originally came to see me 13 years ago complaining of severe lower backache that she had suffered from for 20 years. She had fractured a transverse process on one of her lumbar vertebrae in 1971 which resulted in major back surgery in 1974. The operation had not been successful as she had had to take painkillers ever since.

If you look at the photo to the right you can see a 14cm transverse scar running across her lower back just below the clips at the bottom of the back. When she first came the scar was a keloid scar about 7mm wide and 2mm raised and very red and had been like that for 20 years. Part of the treatment which is not illustrated here is that I passed an electric current along and across the scar and after only four treatments the swelling went down so that the scar became flat and white like a normal scar.

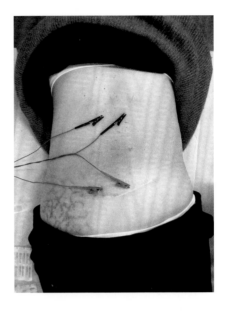

EXAMINATION

Palpation did not reveal any tightness in the lumbar muscles. The pain was primarily on the posterior and lateral sides of the spine itself which felt bony and inflexible.

TREATMENT

1. Applied EA from T12 to L5 on the left and right hand side of the spine along the huatuojiaji points.

2. Added musculoskeletal points with MA: Du-3, Du-4, Bl-40, Ki-4.

3. Added constitutional points with MA: Bl-20, Bl-23, Du-6, all with moxa; Ki-3, St-36, Sp-3, Ren-12, Ren-6.

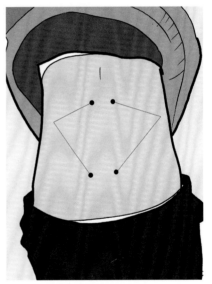

OUTCOME

Although the pain hasn't gone it has diminished to the point where she can live without painkillers. In order to keep the pain at bay she needs a treatment every 6 to 8 weeks.

CASE STUDY

This 44 year old male motorcycle mechanic presented with lower backache on the right side. He also suffered from neck pain on the left side and aching knees. He was generally exhausted, possibly because of the long hours he works - 6 or 7 days a week, plus building work. He also got very hot at night. Part of the problem is that he is 190cm tall and works at a bench which means that he is stooping and bending which exacerbates his neck and back problems. The long periods of standing on concrete floors have affected his knees. All his problems stem from his work situation which I believe has caused or exacerbated his underlying Kidney yin deficiency and Liver qi stagnation with Blood stagnation.

EXAMINATION

Palpation revealed tightness in the quadratus lumborum and longissimus muscles in the right lumbar region. Also tightness and soreness in the levator scapulae muscle on the left side. The knees were not particularly swollen and had no obvious bony changes.

TREATMENT

1. Applied EA from the neck insertion of the levator scapulae muscle to its insertion on the scapula on the left side.

2. Applied EA along the longissimus muscle from T12 to L5 on the right side.

3. Applied EA from the superior border of the quadratus lumborum to the inferior border on the right side.

4. Applied EA from Liv-8 to a point on the lateral side of each leg between GB-33 and GB-34 on the joint line.

5. Added other constitutional points with MA: Bl-18, Bl-23, Du-8, Du-4, Du-3, Ki-10, TH-6, Liv-3, LI-11.

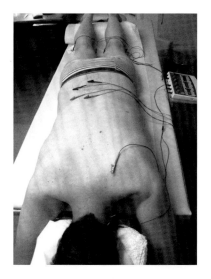

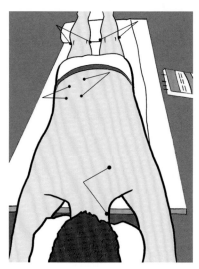

OUTCOME

All his problems diminished considerably apart from his addiction to work which is something he is aware needs addressing; over the last year he has managed to take a couple of holidays that he has really enjoyed so I feel we are making progress. In the meantime, treatment every 6 to 8 weeks keeps him free from pain.

CASE STUDY

This 71 year old patient first came to see me in 1988 complaining of lower backache - which he had suffered from every day for 20 years as a result of a car accident in which he had finished up upside down suspended by his seat belt. At the time of the accident, he was diagnosed with a possible fracture of the lower back and compacted discs. After 4 treatments with MA his backache had almost gone. Over the next 10 years he came back for courses of treatment every 2 to 3 years to keep the back free from pain. By 1999 the treatment was not working; after this I used EA successfully until 2013, at which point the treatment stopped working again. There was a promising brief period where Tung acupuncture seemed to provide a solution but the pain eventually came back. And we decided to stop treatment.

After a 4 year break he decided to come back. The pain had got worse and he was starting to lose the ability to stand up straight. This indicated that the psoas muscles were possibly involved. When he adopted the lunge position there was more tightness on the left side (where he felt the pain) than the right. The lunge position stretches the psoas and so can reveal any excessive tightness in this muscle.

TREATMENT

1. With the patient lying on his right side I applied EA from the huatuojiaji points at L1, L2 and L3 on the left side to the insertion of the psoas muscle (near St-31) at the anterior medial side of the femur on the left side.

2. Added no other musculoskeletal points.

3. Added constitutional points with MA: Bl-20, Bl-23, Du-6, Du-4, Du-3, Ki-3, Sp-3.

OUTCOME

The immediate effect was that he could stand up straight which he was very happy about; his wife said later that he was not hobbling about like an old man anymore. We continued with a further 5 treatments but didn't manage to resolve the underlying long term backache: however, standing up straighter meant that he could walk further with less pain.

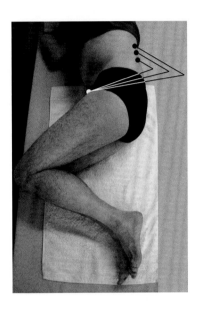

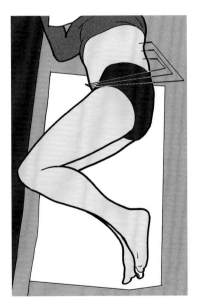

CASE STUDY

This 41 year old woman first came to see me in 2003 with lower backache and sciatica which she had had for 6 weeks. She responded well to MA and was considerably better after 6 treatments. She had tretment once a month over the next year which kept her backache in check. She then stopped treatment.

During the next 6 years her back was fine but eventually the back pain and sciatica returned. Again, treatment seemed to resolve the problem until in 2016 things rapidly deteriorated with seriously herniated discs inferior to L4 and L5 and it was decided because of the severity of the problem to operate. Post-operation she came back for treatment. Although the operation had reduced the acute and severe symptoms considerably, she was still experiencing some back pain which she described as different from her old pain. There was no sciatica now and the only pain she experienced was around the scar tissue at L4 and L5.

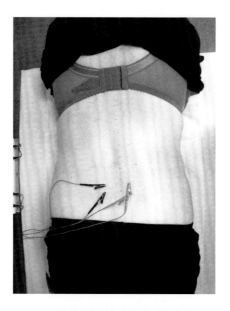

EXAMINATION

Palpation confirmed that the problem was only around L4 and L5; no other lumbar muscles seemed to be implicated.

TREATMENT

1. Applied EA across the spine at L4 and L5.

2. No musculoskeletal points.

3. Added constitutional points with MA: Bl-20, Bl-23, Du-6, Du-4, Du-3, SI-3, Bl-62, Ki-4, Sp-3.

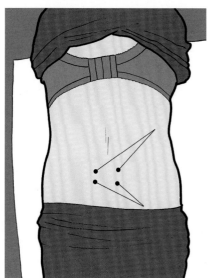

OUTCOME

She has remained pain free with the help of treatments every 6 to 8 weeks.

Hip

12

osteoarthritis, rheumatoid arthritis & bursitis

Osteoarthritis of the hip is a chronic degenerative condition that can affect one hip in isolation without there being any sign of rheumatoid arthritis. An obvious trauma like a fracture or dislocation of the hip can start the process of degenerative changes to the joint. Sometimes osteoarthritis can be triggered by misalignment of the bones in the lumbar sacral region causing the joint to articulate in a different plane and ultimately wear the joint. Heavy lifting or stressful impact exercise can also damage the hip. I remember treating a farmer who had both hips replaced by the time he was 30; in his teens he had spent his summers carrying 100kg sacks.

The condition usually gets worse over a number of years with hip replacement being the only eventual option. However, EA every 4 to 6 weeks can be very helpful in keeping a person pain free for a number of years and thus delaying surgery.

Pain is usually felt after exercise and is often worse at night. Pain is sometimes felt in the groin and down the front of the thigh to the knee; the greater trochanter can be sore when pressed. If this condition is not treated in its early stages then the adaptations that the patient has to make in order to avoid pain when walking can stress other joints, particularly the knee on the opposite leg. There can also be tightening of the lumbar muscles on the same side as the bad hip. This happens because rather than lift the knee and bend the hip joint when walking, the patient will unconsciously lift the pelvis on the side of the bad hip and so avoid the discomfort of moving the hip joint itself. Over a period of time this can result in the quadratus lumborum and spinae erector muscles becoming tight on the side of the bad hip together with the possible complication of sciatica. The gluteus medius and maximus, iliotibial band and piriformis can also become tight. EA both addresses the hip joint specifically and frees up the constricted muscles in the lower back, buttock and leg.

Rheumatoid arthritis is a systemic inflammatory autoimmune disease affecting the joints. Bursitis of the hip is an inflammatory condition of one or both of the bursas of the hip joint. A bursa is a fluid-filled sac that functions as a gliding surface to reduce friction between moving tissues of the body. One bursa covers the greater trochanter, the other is on the medial side of the hip joint.

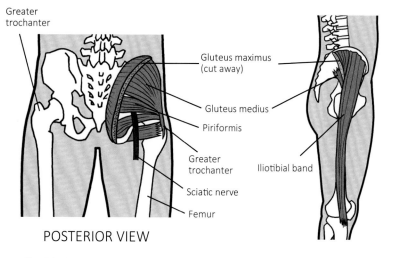

POSTERIOR VIEW

Fig. 12. 1.

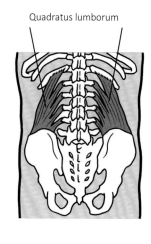

Fig. 12. 2.

Fig. 12. 3.

UNDERLYING STRUCTURES

The muscles of the hip fall into three main groups: the hip muscles, the gluteal muscles and the thigh muscles. Some directly connect to the greater trochanter like the gluteus maximus, gluteus medius and piriformis (Fig. 12. 1).

We should also be aware of the iliotibial band tendon (Fig. 12. 2). At the superior end it splits into two branches: one branch attaches directly to the iliac crest; the other incorporates the tensor fasciae latae and then attaches to the iliac crest. The lower end attaches to the lateral side of the knee.

The muscles of the lumbar region which include the iliocostalis, longissimus and quadratus lumborum also play a significant role in the treatments outlined here (Figs. 12. 3 and 12. 4).

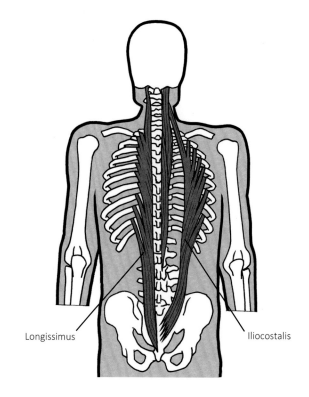

Fig. 12. 4.

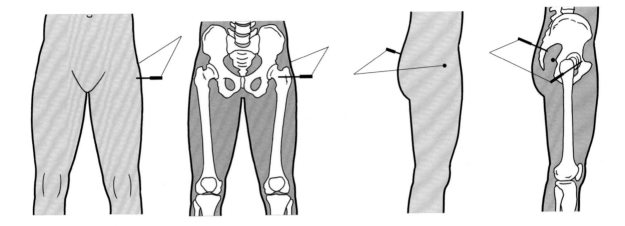

ANTERIOR VIEW   LATERAL VIEW

Basic hip treatment

Palpate the hip, buttock and lower back to ascertain which muscles are involved or have been affected by the hip problem. Begin by pressing firmly on the greater trochanter as this is often sore with osteoarthritis of the hip, then palpate the gluteus maximus and medius, and piriformis - often GB-30 will be tender. Next palpate the iliocostalis, longissimus, quadratus lumborum and iliotibial band.

The purpose of this simple hip treatment is to pass electricity through and around the hip joint.

1 With the patient lying face down, insert a 75mm needle vertically in Bl-54. Insert a second 75mm needle horizontally in a point just anterior to the greater trochanter; it should be parallel to the couch and perpendicular to the side of the leg. Attach EA clips.

2 Needle any other local ashi points with MA.

3 Add musculoskeletal points with MA: GB-30, GB-41.

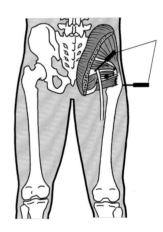

POSTERIOR VIEW

4 Treat constitutional points with MA.

5 Turn on the EA machine, set the frequency to 90/30Hz DD and carefully turn up the intensity to a point where the patient feels a comfortable tingling or pulsing sensation. Treat with EA for 10 to 20 minutes.

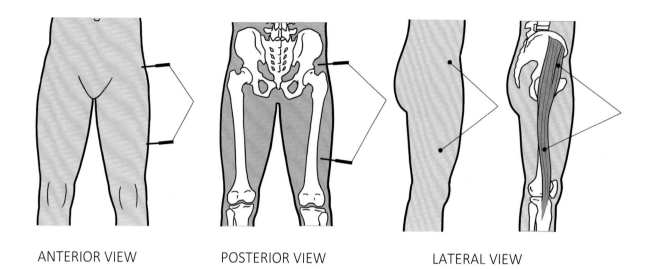

ANTERIOR VIEW   POSTERIOR VIEW   LATERAL VIEW

Iliotibial band treatment

In this treatment we are addressing the iliotibial band which is often tight and sore in people with hip pain. Usually this can be addressed with MA, although in severe chronic cases, EA may be necessary.

1   With the patient lying face down palpate the iliotibial band for any ashi points.

2   Insert a needle at GB-29 and another in any ashi point on the iliotibial band around GB-31. Attach EA clips.

3   Turn on the EA machine, set the frequency to 6/2Hz DD and carefully turn up the intensity to a point where the patient feels a comfortable tingling or pulsing sensation. Treat with EA for 10 to 20 minutes.

NOTE

This treatment can be applied simultaneously to the basic hip treatment.

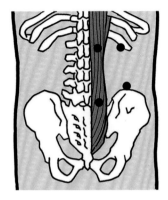 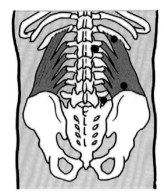 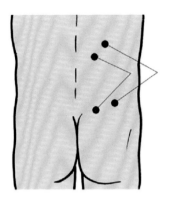

Longissimus & quadratus lumborum treatment

With more chronic hip problems, the quadratus lumborum on the side of the painful hip becomes sore because of the habitual lifting of the pelvis in order to avoid moving the painful hip joint. Eventually this tightening can also affect the longissimus muscle. The tightening of these muscles can complicate the hip problem by provoking back pain and sciatica.

1 Palpate the lumbar region on the same side as the painful hip to establish whether there are ashi points on the longissimus muscle and/or the quadratus lumborum .

2 Insert needles at the superior and inferior aspects of the longissimus and/or quadratus lumborum muscle. Attach EA clips.

3 Needle any other local ashi points with MA.

4 Add musculoskeletal points with MA: Bl-40, Bl-60, GB-34.

5 Treat constitutional points with MA.

6 Turn on the EA machine, set the frequency to 6/2Hz DD and carefully turn up the intensity to a point where the patient feels a comfortable tingling or pulsing sensation. Treat with EA for 10 to 20 minutes.

Bony changes to the posterior of the hip

In severe cases of osteoarthritis of the hip with palpable bony changes, i.e. a thickening of the posterior aspect of the hip joint, apply EA from yaoyan (M-BW-25) to Bl-37 combined with the other hip treatments outlined in this chapter.

CASE STUDY

This 68 year old female presented with lower back pain, osteoarthritis of the left hip, sciatica down the left side, knee pain on the right side and arthritis in her fingers. She found it too painful to lie on her left side at night and had been using a walking stick for a year. She was unable to walk very far without being in considerable pain. She was taking amitriptyline, codeine, clopidogrel, paracetamol, ramipril, simvastatin and tramadol. 20 years previously she had undergone surgery to fuse the spine using rods in the lumbar region. 3 years previously she had suffered a heart attack. From a TCM perspective she has Spleen and Kidney yang deficiency.

EXAMINATION

Palpation revealed tightness and soreness in the longissimus and quadratus lumborum muscles on the left side. There was also soreness on the greater trochanter and tenderness at GB-30(L).

TREATMENT

1. Applied EA from L1 to L5 on the left side.

2. Applied EA from QL1 to QL5 on the left side.

3. Applied EA from Bl-54(L) to the hip point anterior to the left trochanter.

4. Added musculoskeletal points with MA: Bl-40(L), GB-30(L), GB-31(L), GB-41(L).

5. Added constitutional points with MA: Bl-20, Bl-23, Du-6, Du-4, Du-3, Ki-3, Sp-3, St-36, Ren-6, Ren-12.

OUTCOME

After the first treatment there was an immediate reduction in the back pain, sciatica and hip pain. By the 4th treatment she was much improved. Her legs felt lighter and she was walking without a stick.

As treatment progressed she steadily improved. However, the right knee didn't respond to either MA or EA and will probably need surgery.

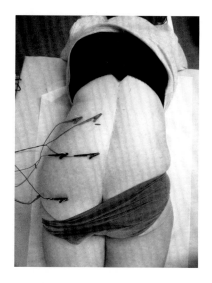

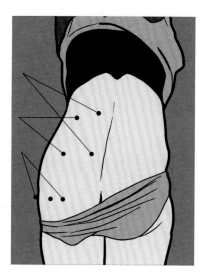

CASE STUDY

This 84 year old woman presented with hip pain, possibly osteoarthritis of the hip: I hesitate to call it osteoarthritis as I had been treating it intermittently for 20 years with long periods of complete relief and no x-rays were taken to confirm the diagnosis. The last episode was 3 years previously when the pain in her right hip was so bad that she was confined to the house. It seemed that hip replacement was going to be the only answer. In addition she was experiencing knee pain on the left side which is not uncommon when the patient tries to adapt their gait to the bad hip. The patient was taking thyroxine 25mcg and BP tablets.

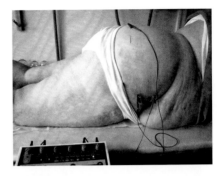

EXAMINATION

Palpation revealed no involvement of the lumbar muscles.

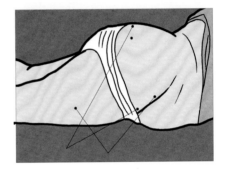

TREATMENT

1. EA from Bl-54(R) to the hip point anterior to the right trochanter.

2. EA from GB-29(R) to an ashi point on the iliotibial band.

3. Added musculoskeletal points with MA: GB-30(R) and GB-41(R).

4. Added constitutional points with MA: Bl-20, Bl-23, Du-6, Du 4, Du-3, Ki-3, Sp-3, St-36.

OUTCOME

After 6 treatments the hip pain was 80% better and she was able to walk a lot further. Over the next 8 months she had 10 more treatments which seem to have resolved the problem completely.

CASE STUDY

This 70 year old woman initially came for treatment for painful knees. The knee problems were a result of Spleen qi deficiency and Kidney yin deficiency with an accumulation of Dampness in the joints and degeneration of the bone. The knees improved considerably and the improvement was maintained by a treatment once every 6 to 8 weeks. Occasionally she would complain of some discomfort in her right hip which would be addressed successfully during the treatment with MA; however, recently, the pain became so bad that she was woken every night. An x-ray revealed that she had fairly severe arthritis in her right hip but not severe enough to operate. We therefore decided to start weekly EA treatments on the hip.

EXAMINATION

On palpation of the spinae erector muscles, I found the longissimus on the right was sore. The lateral side of the trochanter on the right was tender to the touch. The iliotibial band on the right was also sore.

TREATMENT

1. Applied EA from L1 to L5 on the right side of the lower spine.

2. Applied EA from Bl-54(R) to the hip point anterior to the right trochanter.

3. Applied EA from GB-29(R) to GB-31(R).

4. Applied EA from GB-30(R) to GB-41(R). This was experimental and I do not think it was an improvement on my regular hip treatment.

5. No other musculoskeletal points.

6. Added constitutional points with MA: Bl-20, Bl-23, Du-6, Du-4, K-6, LI-11, Sp-6, St-36, Ren-4, Ren-12.

OUTCOME

After the first treatment with EA she was able to sleep through the night pain free. With further treatment her pain was considerably less and she now has a treatment every month.

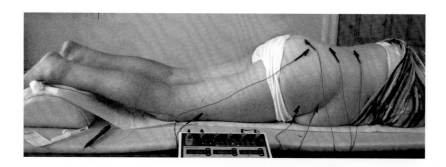

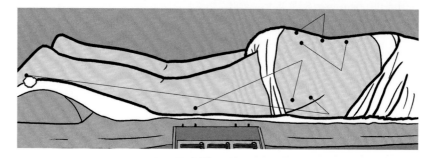

Groin strain

13

A groin strain usually refers to a strain, tear or rupture of one of the adductor muscle tendon attachments to the pubic bone.

A partial rupture of these tendons often leads to them becoming inflamed or to tendinopathy after the initial rupture has healed. Groin strains usually occur when sprinting or changing direction quickly or during rapid movements of the leg against resistance e.g. when kicking a ball. Overstretching the muscle such as in martial arts high kicks can also cause an adductor muscle tear.

Treatment of a groin strain with EA is very similar to treatment of tennis elbow as we are addressing any possible chronic contraction of the muscle - which can cause a reduction in its blood supply - while also addressing the damage to the tendon.

The chronic nature and slow healing of these conditions is probably the result of poor blood supply to the tendon together with continued repetitive use.

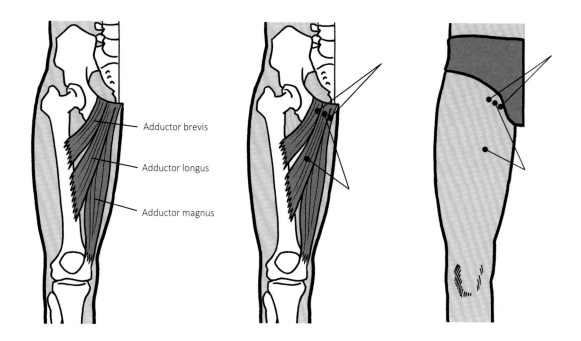

Adductor brevis

Adductor longus

Adductor magnus

UNDERLYING STRUCTURES

The structures relevant to a groin strain are the hip adductors: adductor brevis, adductor longus, adductor magnus, gracilis and pectineus. Any of these groin muscles can be strained but the most commonly affected is the adductor longus.

Groin strain treatment

1 Commence with the patient lying face up with their knees supported. Locate the insertion of the tendon that is painful and then palpate along the related muscle. This may be the adductor brevis, adductor longus, adductor magnus, gracilis or pectineus. Identify any sore or tight spots in the belly of the muscle preferably somewhere halfway along.

2 Insert a needle directly into the affected tendon at its insertion and another needle distal in the body of the muscle and attach one pair of EA clips.

3 Insert 2 needles either side of the tendon and attach another pair of EA clips.

4 Add musculoskeletal channel points with MA according to the channel affected.

5 Add constitutional points with MA.

6 Turn on the EA machine, set the frequencies to 6/2Hz DD along the muscle and 20/6Hz DD across the tendon - if you only have one machine use 6/2Hz for both - and carefully turn up the intensity to a point where the patient feels a comfortable tingling or pulsing sensation. Treat with EA for 10 to 20 minutes.

NOTE

It may be necessary to use at least 50mm needles either side of the tendon insertion in order to go deep enough to make this treatment effective.

CASE STUDY

This 28 year old male presented with a lower back problem on the right hand side radiating down the back of the leg and a groin sprain on the same side. He had been suffering from back problems for 3 years and the groin problem for 4 months. He was a keen footballer and all his problems were worse after playing. His other accompanying signs and symptoms were flat feet, tendency to shin splints and discomfort on the medial sides of his knees. Pulse diagnosis revealed Spleen qi deficiency.

EXAMINATION

Examination of the back revealed sore points along the longissimus muscle in the lumbar spine from L2 to L5 on the right hand side; also tenderness along the quadratus lumborum muscle on the right. The insertion of the adductor longus on the right was sore and there was tenderness along the muscle itself.

TREATMENT

1. With the patient face down, applied EA both from L2(R) to L5(R) and from QL2 to QL8.

2. With the patient face up, applied EA along the adductor longus, placing the first needle into the tendon and the second needle in the muscle above the knee.

3. Applied EA across the adductor longus tendon just inferior to the insertion in the pubic bone.

4. Added musculoskeletal point with MA: GB-34.

5. Added constitutional points with MA: Bl-20, St-36, Sp-3.

OUTCOME

Five treatments resolved the lower back and groin pain, although I suspect that he will be back if he continues to play football.

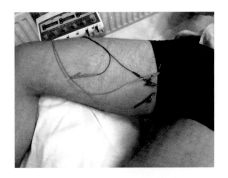
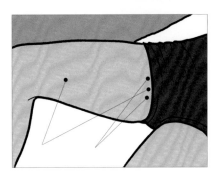

Knee

osteoarthritis, rheumatoid arthritis, cartilage & cruciate ligament problems

14

The downside of being a biped is the stress it puts on our hips and knees. In Elaine Morgan's book *The Scars of Evolution* she hypothesises that we made our leap from ape to human during a long period in the water wading about and swimming, eating high protein food and learning to stand erect. It may be that standing on dry land does not suit our joints. It is interesting to observe that apes do not really stand for long periods but sit or 'walk' on all fours. So maybe cycling, rather than walking or running, might be better for our hips and knees. Anyway, I digress. The knee is one of the most unstable joints in the body, partly because of its position: it has neither the stability the ground provides for the ankle, nor the stability the pelvic muscles provide for the hip joint.

Pain in the knee can arise for a number of reasons.

1. Pain from the muscular insertions around the knee joint.

2. Pain due to damage of the cartilage. Tears in the cartilage can result in pieces of cartilage becoming detached and floating freely in the joint: this can lead to the occasional locking of the joint.

3. Pain caused by tears to the cruciate ligaments, often as the result of injury.

4. Pain caused by rheumatoid arthritis.

5. Pain as a result of osteoarthritis of the knee with degeneration of the bone: this may be due to damage of the cartilage making bone rub on bone.

From a TCM perspective, knee problems can be caused by the Kidneys not nourishing the bones; Spleen deficiency allowing too much fluid to accumulate around the knees causing stiffness; or the Liver not supporting the tendons leading to pain and instability. With knee problems, it is particularly important to address the underlying constitutional weaknesses as well as the musculoskeletal aspects.

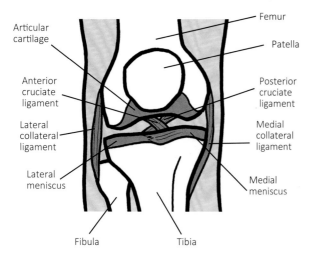

Articular cartilage

Femur

Patella

Anterior cruciate ligament

Posterior cruciate ligament

Lateral collateral ligament

Medial collateral ligament

Lateral meniscus

Medial meniscus

Fibula

Tibia

ANTERIOR VIEW OF THE RIGHT KNEE

UNDERLYING STRUCTURES

The internal structure of the knee joint includes the lateral and medial meniscus, and the posterior and anterior cruciate ligaments. The more external structures include the medial and lateral collateral ligaments. There are many muscles both anterior, posterior and lateral that attach above and below the knee that we will not be discussing here because this particular protocol addresses inflammation and tissue damage in the interior of the knee.

I will however mention the insertions of the hamstrings and calf muscles at the back of the knee that are often sore and may well need treating with MA. I suspect these are often not considered in a standard acupuncture approach.

In terms of treatment we can have a significant influence on knee problems by using MA to release any tight muscles with insertions in the knee. The points that we would use often coincide with local traditional knee points.

I tend to think of EA to the knee, using the following method, as an electrical arthroscopy; obviously it is not possible to get rid of debris from the knee joint but it is possible to stimulate the body's own healing. The aim of this treatment is quite simply to direct the flow of electricity through the joint itself. Over the years I have found this method more successful than applying EA above and below the knee.

There are situations where the patient complains of pain in the bony area lateral or medial to the knee cap. In these situations it is important to track which muscle insertions may be the cause and treat the relevant muscle and insertion with EA .

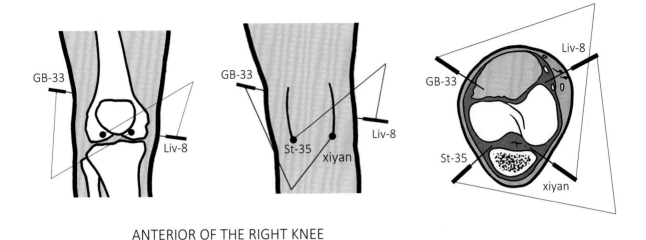

ANTERIOR OF THE RIGHT KNEE

CROSS SECTION OF
THE KNEE JOINT

Knee treatment

1 With the patient lying on their back, place a support under their knees. Raising the knees allows for a deeper and easier insertion into xiyan and St-35.

2 Insert needles in GB-33, Liv-8, St-35 and xiyan. Attach one pair of EA clips from St-35 to Liv-8 and another pair from GB-33 to xiyan.

3 Needle any other local ashi points with MA.

4 Add supplementary points with MA according to the underlying patterns and channels affected e.g. GB-34, Ki-3, Ki-10, Liv-7, Liv-8, St-34, St-36, St-41, Sp-5, Sp-9, Liv-8.

5 Treat constitutional points with MA.

6 Turn on the EA machine, set the frequency to 90/30Hz DD and carefully turn up the intensity to a point where the patient feels a comfortable tingling or pulsing sensation. Treat with EA for 10 to 20 minutes.

NOTE

I have tried applying EA using points posterior to GB-33 and Liv-8 but this seems to cause unpleasant sensations running down the leg. I have also tried applying EA from GB-34 to Sp-10 and Sp-9 to St-34 simultaneously with the treatment outlined here, but have not found it to be more effective.

CASE STUDY

This 71 year old male self-employed gardener presented with osteo or rheumatoid arthritis of the knees that had been gradually getting worse over the previous 10 years. Pain was worse after walking and when the weather was cold and damp. Underlying constitutional issues were some Kidney deficiency and Blood stasis.

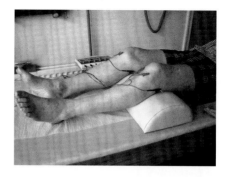

EXAMINATION

On examination there was no swelling of the knees but some thickening and enlargement of the joint; otherwise he was generally fit and well for his age. He was keen to continue work and avoid knee replacements.

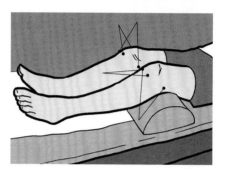

TREATMENT

1. Applied EA from Liv-8(L&R) to St-35(L&R).
2. Applied EA from GB-33(L&R) to xiyan(L&R).
3. No musculoskeletal points.
4. Added constitutional points with MA: Ht-5, Ki-3, P-6 and Liv-3.

OUTCOME

He was very responsive to treatment and after the 4th treatment was able to walk for an hour without pain which was three times further than previously. After the 5th treatment mobility was 50% better and pain was 25% less. After the 8th treatment he could walk even further and had stopped wearing his knee supports. He has now been coming for 4 years once a month and has maintained his improvement. The patient's feedback about the treatment was that although MA was helpful, EA was more effective and longer lasting.

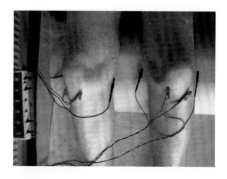

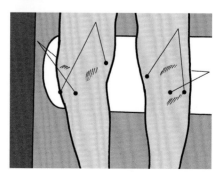

Achilles tendonitis

15

Achilles tendonitis is a painful condition of the Achilles tendon which attaches the calf muscle to the calcaneus. With this condition there can be burning and swelling along the tendon for 2 to 8cm proximal to the heel which tend to be worse when walking and running. This condition can make the skin on your heel feel overly warm to the touch. Sometimes friction can be felt when palpating the tendon and moving the ankle at the same time. There can also be pain in the calf muscle, and a limited range of movement, particularly when dorsi-flexing the foot.

This condition can be caused by overuse and is prevalent in athletes, especially those competing in sports that involve lunging or jumping. It can also be caused by a strain induced injury. Some patients report that stressful situations in their lives correlate with the onset of this condition. The Achilles tendon, like all tendons, has a poor blood supply; this means that any damage or degeneration may be slow to heal.

UNDERLYING STRUCTURES

The Achilles tendon, also known as the calcaneal tendon, is the thickest tendon in the human body. It attaches the gastrocnemius and soleus muscles to the calcaneus bone.

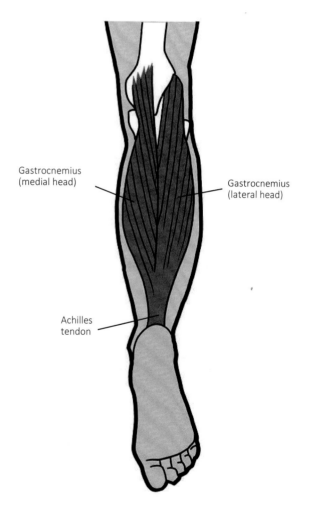

Gastrocnemius
(medial head)

Gastrocnemius
(lateral head)

Achilles
tendon

Achilles tendon treatment

1 With the patient lying face down and their legs supported under the ankles, palpate the Achilles tendon for ashi points .

2 Insert a needle 1cm deep in the back of the Achilles tendon just superior to the calcaneous (Fig. 15.1). Insert another needle approximately 3 tsun superior to this needle. Connect these two points with one pair of EA clips.

3 Insert needles either side of the Achilles tendon where it is sore. 2 or 3 pairs are sufficient. The needles don't have to penetrate the tendon and can be inserted just beneath the skin. Attach the EA clips in pairs across the tendon.

4 Add musculoskeletal points with MA: Bl-54, GB-34.

5 Add constitutional points with MA.

6 Turn on the EA machine, set the frequency to 20/6Hz DD and carefully turn up the intensity to a point where the patient feels a comfortable tingling or pulsing sensation. Treat with EA for 10 to 20 minutes.

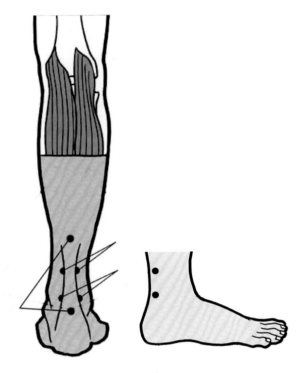

Fig. 15.1

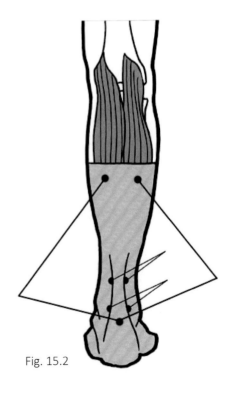

Fig. 15.2

Achilles tendon treatment
involving the gastrocnemius

1   With the patient lying face down and their legs supported under the ankles, palpate the medial and lateral gastrocnemius muscles and the Achilles tendon for ashi points.

2   If you find ashi points in the gastrocnemius muscles, place one needle in both the lateral and medial gastrocnemius (Fig. 15.2). Insert a needle 1cm in the back of the Achilles tendon just superior to the calcaneous. Attach 2 pairs of EA clips from the gastrocnemius points to the Achilles tendon point, making sure that you have the same colour clips on the tendon point.

3   Insert needles either side of the Achilles tendon where it is sore. 2 or 3 pairs are sufficient. The needles don't have to penetrate the tendon and can be inserted just beneath the skin.

4   Add musculoskeletal points with MA: Bl-54, GB-34.

5   Add constitutional points with MA.

6   Turn on the EA machine, set the frequencies to 6/2Hz DD along the muscle and 20/6Hz DD across the tendon - if you only have one machine use 6/2Hz for both - and carefully turn up the intensity to a point where the patient feels a comfortable tingling or pulsing sensation. Treat with EA for 10 to 20 minutes.

CASE STUDY

This 46 year old woman, who was a keen kickboxer, presented with multiple muscle strains around her body. These included tendonitis in her left Achilles tendon, a chronic twisted right ankle, a pulled muscle on the medial side of her lower left leg around Sp-6, sprained wrists, a pulled muscle in her left shoulder and golfer's elbow in her left elbow. Other symptoms included a chronic sore throat, breathlessness on exertion and thick rubbery brown mucus. From a TCM perspective she was suffering from long term Lung and Spleen qi deficiency with an accumulation of Phlegm and probably Lingering Pathogens. In this example we are just going to look at the Achilles tendonitis treatment.

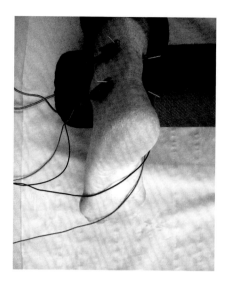

EXAMINATION

The ankle was a little swollen and the Achilles tendon was tender when pinched from the sides.

TREATMENT

1. Applied EA diagonally across the Achilles tendon with 2 pairs of EA leads.

2. No other local musculoskeletal needles were added.

3. Added constitutional points with MA: Bl-13, Bl-20, Du-6, Lu-5, Lu-7, St-40, Sp-6, Sp-9, Ren-12.

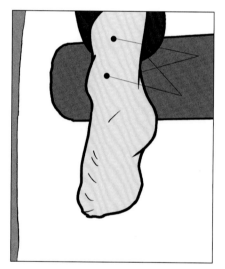

OUTCOME

The Achilles problem was resolved after 5 treatments; the strained muscle on the medial side of the left leg and the right ankle sprain also improved using EA. However, the left shoulder and elbow problem did not respond at all.

Her phlegm turned from brown to clear after a few acupuncture treatments. I am continuing treatment with Chinese herbs to resolve phlegm. I think that the persistence of her muscular strain problems were caused by her underlying constitutional weaknesses.

Plantar fasciitis

16

Plantar fasciitis (also known as policeman's heel) is a painful condition of the base of the foot, particularly the heel. The heel pain is usually unilateral, and is usually worse after periods of rest e.g. when first putting weight on the foot in the morning. The causes of this condition are not entirely clear, but obesity, injury, excessive exercise and long periods of standing can be contributory factors.

It is characterised by pain and soreness at the base of the foot where the plantar fascia attaches to the medial tubercle of the plantar aspect of the calcaneus although it can affect the back or sides of the heel. The plantar fascia is a thick fibrous band of connective tissue that originates from the medial tubercle and anterior aspect of the calcaneal tuberosity: from here the fascia extends along the sole of the foot before inserting into the base of the toes thus supporting the arch of the foot. Some sources suggest that this is not a problem with the fascia itself but is a tendon injury involving the flexor digitorum brevis muscle located above the plantar fascia.

Most cases of plantar fasciitis resolve themselves in time with appropriate rest. One of the reasons why plantar fasciitis can become chronic is because it is difficult to avoid using your feet, thus not giving the tissue an opportunity to heal.

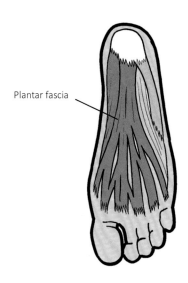

Plantar fascia

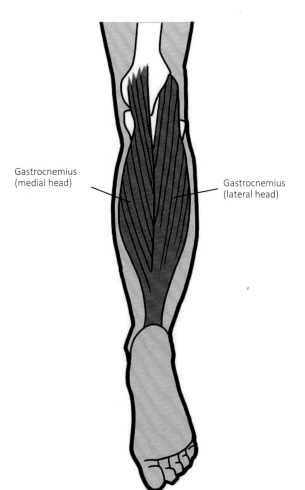

Gastrocnemius
(medial head)

Gastrocnemius
(lateral head)

UNDERLYING STRUCTURES

There are two main structures to take note of with this condition: the gastrocnemius muscles and the plantar fascia that runs from the toes to the calcaneus. If either of these are tight it can cause or exacerbate plantar fasciitis.

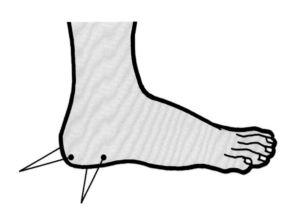
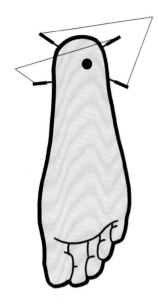

Plantar fasciitis treatment

1 With the patient lying face down on the couch and the ankle supported, palpate the base of the heel and mark any points of soreness. In order to do this, it is necessary to press quite hard so I suggest you use the second finger joint method to palpate as outlined on page 67. This method provides a small enough and hard enough surface to identify the points of tenderness accurately.

2 Palpate the back of the gastrocnemius muscles and needle any ashi points with MA.

3 Next palpate the area anterior to the heel where the fascia runs distally to the toes to identify any sore spots. As needling these points can be painful, I avoid doing so unless the basic treatment is not working. As with any potentially painful points, press the guide tube firmly onto the skin before inserting the needles to minimise discomfort.

4 Insert 15mm needles, two at the lateral side of the heel and two at the medial side, at the junction of the soft and hard skin. They should be positioned so that if a line was drawn between them they would form a cross bisecting the tender point in the heel. As the insertion of the four needles can be painful, it is unnecessary to cause further discomfort by trying to elicit deqi. Attach two pairs of leads so that the current runs diagonally through the heel, with the two currents intersecting at the painful point.

5 Treat constitutional points with MA.

6 Turn on the EA machine, set the frequency to 20/6Hz DD and carefully turn up the intensity to a point where the patient feels a comfortable tingling or pulsing sensation. Treat with EA for 10 to 20 minutes.

CASE STUDY

This 43 year old male financial advisor presented with the worst plantar fasciitis that I have ever seen. His right foot was so painful that when he arrived home from work in the evening he had to remove his shoes and walk on his toes. It was impossible for him to contemplate lowering his heel onto an uncarpeted floor. The condition was affecting his family life because he was not able to run around with his young children. From a TCM perspective his main problem was Heart and Kidney yin deficiency.

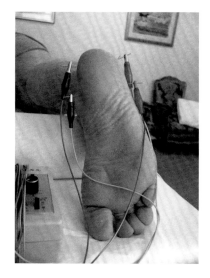

EXAMINATION

On examination of the heel there was one spot that was particularly sore, slightly lateral to the centre of the heel. There did not seem to be any tightness or tenderness in the calf muscles or around the ankle.

TREATMENT

1. Applied EA using two pairs of EA clips diagonally across the heel with the electricity from each pair crossing at the point of tenderness.

2. No other musculoskeletal points.

3. Added constitutional points with MA: Bl-15, Bl-23, Du-14, Ht-6, Ki-6, Ren-14, Ren-4.

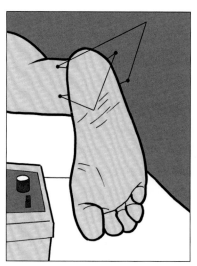

OUTCOME

The improvement was dramatic; the pain abated and after the 4th treatment he spent the weekend laying a patio with no ill effects! And his children were no doubt happy to have a fully mobile dad back.

CASE STUDY

This 67 year old woman presented with plantar fasciitis in her right heel that she had suffered from for two months. She had had carpal tunnel syndrome and migraines in the past, and had experienced constipation and flatulence throughout her life. Her other chronic symptom was irritable bladder with frequent urination at night. From a Chinese perspective she was suffering from Kidney qi deficiency and Liver qi stagnation.

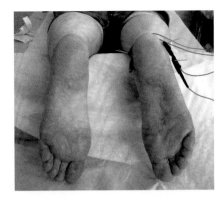

EXAMINATION

Examination of the foot and leg revealed tender spots on the heel of the right foot but no soreness or tightness in the calf muscles.

TREATMENT

1. Applied EA using two pairs of EA clips diagonally across the heel with the electricity from each pair crossing at the point of tenderness.

2. No other musculoskeletal points.

3. Added constitutional points with MA: Bl-18, Bl-23, Du-4, Ki-3, TH-6, GB-34, Liv-3.

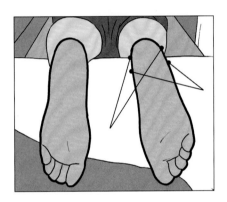

OUTCOME

After the 2nd treatment the pain was 70% better and after the 4th treatment the pain was gone.

Scar tissue

17

Scar tissue is the result of a wound healing. It can be unsightly and even dangerous e.g. a keloid cyst that continues to grow. During the healing process collagen is used to repair the damaged tissue. However, in scar tissue, instead of the random criss-cross pattern of normal tissue, there is a pronounced pattern in one direction which reduces its functional quality.

Various types of scar have been identified. Although each type is composed of collagen, it is the over-expression of collagen that gives each its own characteristics. Types of scar tissue:

ATROPHIC
This occurs when some of the underlying structures supporting the skin are lost, giving the scar a sunken appearance.

HYPERTROPHIC
The raised red areas of a hypertrophic scar are the result of an overproduction of collagen, but can also be due to infection or excessive tension in the scar.

KELOID
This again is caused by an excessive growth of collagen but occurs outside the wound area. Although usually benign, it can be unsightly, itchy and painful.

STRETCH MARKS
Stretch marks, also called striae gravidarum, are caused by excessive stretching of the skin resulting in scars. These can develop during pregnancy or rapid weight gain.

Scars that respond well to EA are: firstly, new scars (treating the scar fairly soon after a hip operation, for example, will facilitate circulation, reduce inflammation and improve healing); secondly, hypertrophic and keloid scars. Scars that are sunken and flaccid do not respond so well because clearing excess tissue is easier than building up tissue.

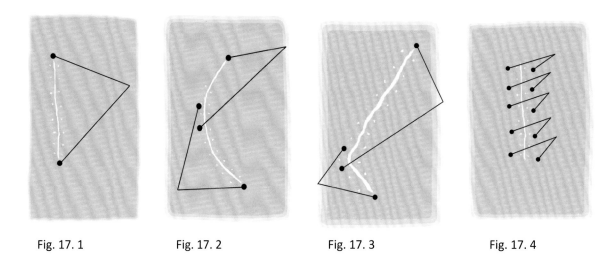

Fig. 17. 1   Fig. 17. 2   Fig. 17. 3   Fig. 17. 4

Scar treatment

As you can see from the diagrams above, the position of the needles and the route of the electrical current are very important. Electricity takes the shortest route from A to B. With a straight scar you simply place a needle at each end of the scar and conduct the electricity in a straight line from one end to the other (Fig. 17. 1). With a curved or irregular-shaped scar you need to divide it into a series of straight lines (Figs. 17. 2 and 17. 3).

Another way of treating scar tissue is to place the needles either side of the scar and then conduct the electricity across the scar in pairs (Fig. 17. 4).

It is important that the needles are inserted only to the same depth as the scar itself. This can be estimated by the type of operation as well as its location. Generally speaking it is not necessary to place the needles in the scar itself to get good results which is fortunate as often the scar tissue can be quite tough making penetration with the needles difficult. Nonetheless, as treatment progresses and the scar tissue becomes softer, it is possible to place the needles in the scar which can enhance the treatment further. Use 90/30Hz DD.

Adding other local, distal and constitutional points can also improve the effectiveness of this treatment.

Unusual & difficult cases

18

This section of the book is devoted to unusual and difficult cases and illustrates that EA is not just effective for musculoskeletal problems. Most of these cases have not been replicated, so it is impossible to know whether the treatments would work on patients with similar problems. However, they do show how important it is to think creatively about difficult cases that are not responding to treatment. This usually involves standing back, reassessing the problem, and looking at it from a new perspective and not limiting yourself to what you believe to be the case. Meticulous questioning of the patient may reveal facts that you might have missed earlier. Just because the consultant thinks that tingling in a patient's hands is caused by the obvious degeneration of the discs in the neck, it does not mean they do not have carpal tunnel syndrome as well!

ACOUSTIC NEUROMA

This 49 year old female presented with an acoustic neuroma (a benign tumour) growing in the right middle ear. It had been diagnosed 18 months previously and was 0.8mm. It was scanned regularly to check if it was growing and, if so, how quickly. The pressure of the tumour on her facial nerves was causing her mouth to stay in a fixed grin on one side which she had to correct manually by pulling her mouth down. Her eye and mouth twitched involuntarily. There was also a constant pulling sensation in the muscles of her face. She complained of tinnitus, a sensation of pressure in her head, and the beginnings of carpal tunnel syndrome. From a TCM perspective she was suffering from Kidney yang deficiency.

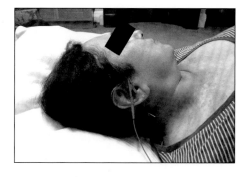

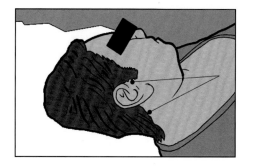

Although the initial treatments with acupuncture and Chinese herbal medicine reduced the tinnitus (and the excessive urination and coldness from which she had also been suffering), her facial symptoms remained the same. I therefore decided to try EA as follows.

TREATMENT

1. Applied EA from SI-19(R) to GB-20(R).

2. Added constitutional points with MA: Ki-3, TH-5, GB-20, GB-43, Liv-3, Ren-6, yintang.

OUTCOME

After 6 treatments all the eye and mouth symptoms ceased even though scans revealed that the tumour was still continuing to grow. At the time of writing the patient is still coming for treatment once a month with no return of her symptoms. It would seem that surgery is the only eventual solution to this problem but at the moment both the patient and her doctor are unwilling to take this step and the symptoms are being controlled.

CALF PAIN

This 62 year old female presented with severe pain in her calves. Even after walking short distances, the pain could keep her awake all night. An MRI scan revealed degenerative changes to the bottom three lumbar discs. She had suffered with back pain for many years although recently the pain had gone. It was thought that the leg problem was due to nerves in the lower back being trapped.

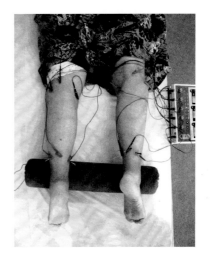

From a TCM perspective she was suffering from Kidney yin deficiency and Spleen qi deficiency. Initially, treating back shu points, distal points and huatuojiaji points in the lumbar region improved the condition to a limited degree. However, I was not convinced that the pain in the calf muscles was caused by nerve problems in the back. This woman had spent many years standing in a factory which I believed had resulted in localised Blood stagnation in the calves. I recalled a story about Doctor Shen identifying Blood stagnation in a particular muscle group as a patient's main problem.

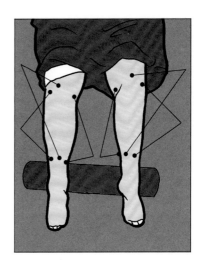

TREATMENT

Applied EA along the full length of the calf muscles, using three pairs of EA clips on each leg.

OUTCOME

The result of this was a dramatic improvement in her pain levels and she was able to walk a couple of miles without being up all night in pain. With more treatment she made further progress. This case demonstrates that sometimes we can be too holistic in our approach and miss severe localised stagnation.

DUPUYTREN'S CONTRACTURE

This 54 year old man presented with the beginning stages of Dupuytren's contracture with thickening of the tissue in the palm of the left hand resulting in nodules and contraction of the tendons, particularly in the 2nd and 3rd fingers. The patient also presented with a plethora of other problems, including long term Pathogenic Factor remaining.

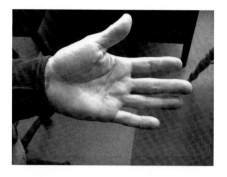

TREATMENT

1. Inserted needles at each end of the two bands of thickened tissue on the palm, in line with the 2nd and 3rd fingers. Attached two pairs of EA clips and applied EA.

2. Inserted a needle in the nodule on the 2nd finger tendon and one in the nodule on the 3rd finger tendon. Attached a pair of EA clips and applied EA.

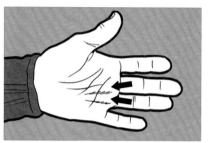

OUTCOME

I treated the patient once a week for 8 weeks by which point the nodules and thickened tissue had dispersed. That was 8 years ago. This year, the tissue began to thicken once more; I repeated the treatment and the nodules and thickened tissue dispersed once again.

I have performed this treatment once before with long term remission. I have also treated Dupuytren's contracture in its more advanced stage with no success at all. So the important lesson to learn here is that treatment in the early stages is essential.

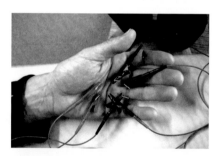

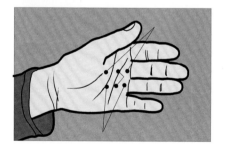

HERPES ZOSTER

This 67 year old man presented with shingles on the right side of his upper back, armpit and chest. He had had the condition for 3 weeks and taken a course of antiviral drugs. The spots had abated but he was still in considerable pain. The underlying cause of his problem was Damp Heat in the Liver. This was probably the result of the 14 pints of beer he consumed per week.

EXAMINATION

The upper back on the right hand side from T5 to T11 was tender to the touch. The huatuojiaji region from C7(R) to T11(R) was tight.

TREATMENT 1 (Fig. 1)

1. Applied EA from C7(R) to T11(R) and needled alternate huatuojiaji points in between with MA.
2. Added constitutional points with MA: Bl-18, Bl-20, Du-9, Du-6, TH-6, Liv-2, LI-11, Sp-9, St-36, Ren-12.

OUTCOME

The pain in the back, chest and armpit was less severe.

TREATMENTS 2 and 3 (Figs. 1 and 2)

1. Applied EA from C7(R) to T11(R) and needled alternate huatuojiaji points in between with MA as in treatment 1. (Fig. 1)
2. Applied 4 pairs of EA leads from the thoracic huatuojiaji points on the right hand side of the spine to the side of the torso following the line of the dermatomes. (Fig. 2)

3. Added constitutional points with MA: Bl-18, Bl-20, Du-9, Du-6, TH-6, Liv-2, LI-11, Sp-9, St-36, Ren-12.

OUTCOME

The pain in the back stopped completely and the pain in the chest and armpit diminished further.

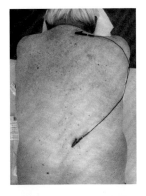

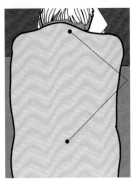

Fig. 1

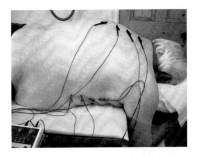

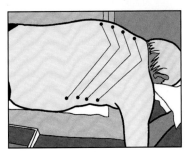

Fig. 2

TREATMENT 4

1. With the patient lying on his front, applied 4 pairs of EA leads from the thoracic huatuojiaji points on the right hand side of the spine to the side of the torso following the line of the dermatomes (Fig. 2).

2. With the patient lying on his back, applied 4 pairs of EA leads from just medial to the sternum to the side of the body (Fig. 3).

3. Added constitutional points with MA: Bl-18, Bl-20, Du-9, Du-6, TH-6, Liv-2, LI-11, Sp-9, St-36, Ren-12.

OUTCOME

The painful area in the chest became smaller, but the pain in the armpit had not improved any further.

TREATMENTS 5 and 6 (Fig. 4)

1. Applied 4 pairs of EA leads across the chest over the now reduced area of pain.
2. Applied 3 pairs of EA leads across the armpit.
3. Added constitutional points with MA: Bl-18, Bl-20, Du-9, Du-6, TH-6, Liv-2, LI-11, Sp-9, St-36, Ren-12.

OUTCOME

The chest and armpit pain was now reduced to an occasional itch and we discontinued treatment.

WARNING Don't try this treatment in the cardiac region on the left side of the chest.

I have treated a number of cases of postherpetic neuralgia which can be severe and debilitating. If this problem is not dealt with effectively in the early stages then the nerves can be permanently damaged, resulting in chronic pain. The EA approach to this problem is to apply EA from the nerve roots on the spine, following the dermatomes diagonally around the torso, and then address localised areas of pain. Although pain may initially be coming from the nerve roots in the spine, I think that the chronic pain that develops is nerve damage in localised areas.

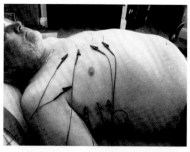

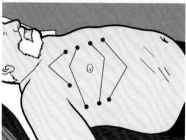

Fig. 3

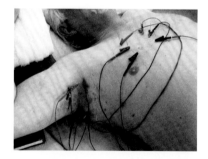

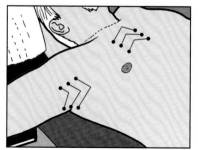

Fig. 4

ITCHING PALM

This 65 year old female presented with a variety of symptoms after a mastectomy for breast cancer with extensive reconstructive surgery using tissue from her back. She had started the menopause two years prior to the surgery. When she arrived she was suffering from neck pain, back pain, hip pain, hot flushes and headaches. She was taking Arimidex. With treatment most of these symptoms were resolved.

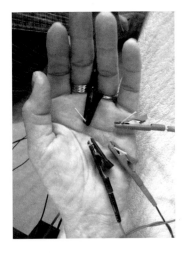

However, she was also suffering from an area of itchy, thick, dry skin in the centre of the palm of her left hand that had bothered her for 5 years. The itching had started immediately after she had come round from her operation, and had been unremitting ever since. Although the condition was nothing compared to everything else she had had, it was a considerable irritation. She was constantly trying creams and various plasters, covering it and not covering it, etc.

Due to the thickening of the skin and obvious localised inflammation I decided to vigorously move qi and Blood with EA.

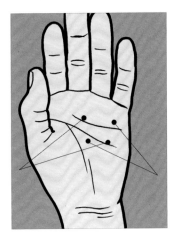

TREATMENT
1. Placed four needles in a square surrounding the area and applied EA diagonally across the thickened skin.

OUTCOME
After one treatment, the itching stopped completely. I repeated the treatment once more and that was 18 months ago. Since then the area has completely healed. Cases like this make me realise that stagnation can occur in very small areas that need addressing locally and that remarkable results can be achieved.

JAW CLENCHING

This 38 year old woman presented with tight, painful jaw muscles from habitual clenching. She was unable to open her mouth fully and the jaw clicked. This problem had persisted for a number of years and was getting worse. She was also suffering from daily headaches on her temples and the top of her head. Her underlying constitution was Spleen qi deficiency with Liver qi stagnation.

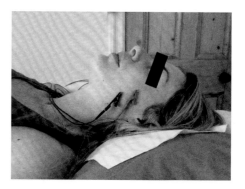

TREATMENT

1. Applied EA from St-6 to St-7 on both sides.
2. Added constitutional points with MA: B-20, B-21. Du-6, Liv-2, GB-20, GB-43, Sp-3, St-36, Ren-12, yintang.

OUTCOME

After the first 2 treatments with MA her headaches abated. Although the jaw pain improved, it was not until I used EA directly on the jaw muscles them-selves that there was a dramatic change and she was able to open her mouth completely.

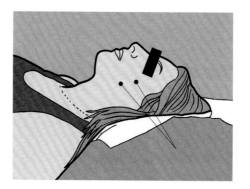

TOOTH PAIN

This 42 year old female presented with chronic tooth pain in the upper and lower jaw which she had been suffering from for 4 years. She was taking amitriptyline and nortriptyline to control the pain. The problem had occurred after a routine filling in her lower jaw. Despite having the filling replaced, the pain was the same. CT scans revealed no possible cause of the pain. Other symptoms included reflux and hot flushes. From a TCM perspective she was suffering from Kidney yin deficiency with Empty Heat. Although MA reduced the flushes by the 4th treatment, there was no improvement in the pain, despite using local and distal points. After also trying auricular acupuncture with no success, I decided by the 5th treatment to use EA.

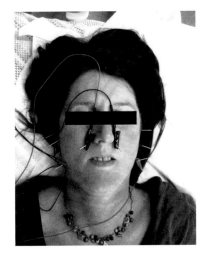

TREATMENT

1. Applied EA from LI-20(L) to TH17(R).

2. Applied EA from LI-20(R) to TH17(L).

3. Applied EA from Si-18(L) to St-6(R).

4. Applied EA from Si-18(R) to St-6(L).

5. Then applied EA from LI-20(L) to St-6(R).

6. And applied EA from LI-20(R) to St-6(L).

7. Added channel points with MA: LI-4, St-44.

8. Added constitutional points with MA: Lu-7, Ki-6, Ren-4.

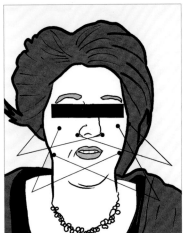

OUTCOME

After 4 treatments of EA she was pain free. She now comes once every 6 to 8 weeks and remains pain free but if she leaves treatment any longer the pain returns.

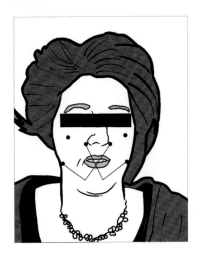

Bibliography

Chan Gunn, C. (1989) The Treatment of Chronic Pain. New York: Churchill Livingstone.

Deadman, P., Al-Khafaji, M., Baker, K. (1998) A Manual of Acupuncture. Hove: Journal of Chinese Medicine Publications.

Gyer, G., Michael, J., Tolson, B. (2016) Dry Needling for Manual Therapists. London: Singing Dragon.

Johnson, I. (2014) Transcutaneous Electrical Nerve Stimulation (TENS). Oxford: Oxford University Press.

Keown, D. (2014) The Spark in the Machine. London: Singing Dragon.

Legge, D. (1997) Close to the Bone. Woy Woy: Sydney College Press.

Maciocia, G. (2006) The Channels of Acupuncture. Philadelphia: Churchill Livingstone.

Maciocia, G. (1994) The Practice of Chinese Medicine. New York: Churchill Livingstone.

Mayor, D. F. (2007) Electroacupuncture. A practical manual and resource. Edinburgh: Churchill Livingstone.

Morgan, E. (1990) The Scars of Evolution. London: Souvenir Press.

Peilin, S. (2002) The Treatment of Pain with Chinese Herbs and Acupuncture. Edinburgh: Churchill Livingstone.

Simons, D. G., Travell, J. G. (1998) Myofascial Pain and Dysfunction: The Trigger Point Manual: Volume 1: Upper Half of Body. Philadelphia: Lippincott Williams and Wilkins.

Simons, D. G., Travell, J. G. (1992) Myofascial Pain and Dysfunction: The Trigger Point Manual: Volume 2: The Lower Extremities. Philadelphia: Lippincott Williams and Wilkins.

Wesley, J. (1760) The Desideratum: or, electricity made plain and useful by a lover of mankind and common sense. Manchester: Gale ECCO.

Biography

Stephen Lee studied five element acupuncture at the College of Traditional Acupuncture in Leamington Spa UK in the early 80s and then studied TCM with Giovanni Maciocia, Peter Deadman, Julian Scott and Vivien Brown in London.

He studied and worked in the acupuncture outpatients department of Nanjing College of Chinese Medicine in China in 1987. In 1991 he completed a 2 year course in Chinese herbal medicine at the School of Chinese Medicine in London with Giovanni Maciocia, Michael McIntyre and Dr Song Ke. He has also completed courses in musculoskeletal acupuncture, electroacupuncture, Master Tung and Dr Tan acupuncture and also gynaecology including infertility.

He has been teaching workshops on electroacupuncture for musculoskeletal problems at the College of Integrated Chinese Medicine and the Northern College of Acupuncture since 2009.

He was a council member and editor of the Register of Chinese Medicine Journal from 2001 to 2006.

Stephen Lee is a member of the BAcC (British Acupuncture Council) and the RCHM (Register of Chinese Herbal Medicine).